# LANGUAGE, INTERACTION AND FRONTOTEMPORAL DEMENTIA

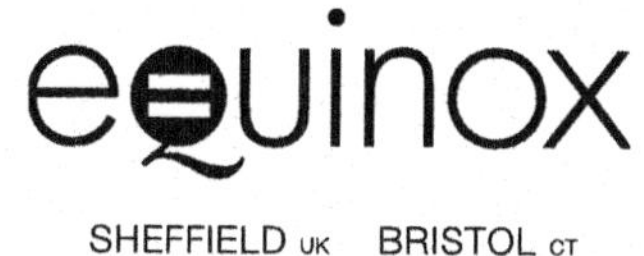

# Language, Interaction and Frontotemporal Dementia

## Reverse Engineering the Social Mind

Edited by

Andrea W. Mates, Lisa Mikesell
and Michael Sean Smith

Published by Equinox Publishing Ltd.

UK: Unit S3, Kelham House, 3 Lancaster Street, Sheffield, South Yorkshire S3 8AF

USA: ISD, 70 Enterprise Drive, Bristol, CT 06010

www.equinoxpub.com

Paperback edition published 2013



British Library Cataloguing-in-Publication Data
A catalogue record for this book is available from the British Library

Library of Congress Cataloging-in-Publication Data

Language, interaction and frontotemporal dementia : reverse engineering the social mind / edited by Andrea W. Mates, Lisa Mikesell and Michael Sean Smith.
    p. cm.
Includes bibliographical references and index.
ISBN 978-1-84553-434-9 (hb)
ISBN 978-1-78179-039-7 (pb)
1.  Language and languages--Physiological aspects. 2. Neurolinguistics. 3.  Dementia--Pathophysiology.  I. Mates, Andrea W. II. Mikesell, Lisa. III. Smith, Michael Sean.  QP399.L373 2010
    612.8'25—dc22
                        2009022812

Typeset and edited by Queenston Publishing, Hamilton, Canada.
Printed in Great Britain

# CONTENTS

# Acknowledgements

This book represents one arm of work in a multi-disciplinary project led by Drs. Alan Page Fiske and Mario Mendez. Jill Shapira provided extensive support and encouragement particularly in the early days as the ethnographies were being collected. The scholars in the other arms of the project are too many to enumerate here, but we would like to particularly highlight the contributions of Sabrina Pagano and Matthew Gervais. Charles Goodwin's focus on embodiment in interaction has influenced both how we analyze and present our data, and John Schumann's passion for the brain and language has been a constant source of inspiration for us. We are grateful to each of these people and their substantial support along the way.

The project has received invaluable seed grants from the UCLA Faculty Senate and the Association for Frontotemporal Dementia. As these chapters were being developed, five were presented at Language, Culture, and Mind 3 in Odense, Denmark. We thank the organizers of Language, Culture, and Mind 3, Olga Yokoyama, Chair of Applied Linguistics, UCLA; Alessandro Duranti, Chair of Anthropology, UCLA; Timothy Stowell, Dean of Humanities, UCLA; and Claudia Mitchell-Kernan, Vice-Chancellor of Graduate Studies, UCLA for their generous financial support which allowed the papers to be presented. We received remarkably incisive feedback from talk attendees whom we would also like to thank.

# Contributors

**Netta Avineri** is currently a doctoral student in Applied Linguistics at the University of California, Los Angeles (UCLA). She earned her Master's degree in Applied Linguistics from UCLA in 2007. Her research interests include ethnography of communication, discourse analysis, institutional talk, and question and response design. She is a recipient of a 2007 UCLA Eugene V. Cota-Robles Fellowship.

**Alan Page Fiske** is a psychological social anthropologist and professor of Anthropology at UCLA. He is author of Structures of Social Life (Free Press, 1991), where he outlined relational models theory, which he continues to explore and develop. He is currently writing a book on the semiotic systems that people use to constitute, coordinate, cognize, communicate, and culturally transmit each of the four fundamental types of social relationships.

**Anna Dina L. Joaquin** received her MA in Applied Linguistics from the University of California, Los Angeles, where she is currently a doctoral candidate. Her interests include the socialization and neurobiology of culture, language and interaction, first and second language acquisition, and discourse analysis. She is a co-author of The Interactional Instinct: The Evolution and Acquisition of Language with four of her colleagues. She is the recipient of a 2005 UCLA Eugene V. Cota-Robles Fellowship.

**Andrea Mates** received her PhD in Applied Linguistics at the University of California, Los Angeles (UCLA). Her primary research interest lies in the neurobiology of language use and language learning. While at UCLA, she co-authored The Interactional Instinct: The Evolution and Acquisition of Language. She also worked on two multi-method research teams; one examining everyday functioning in frontotemporal dementia, and another testing the ecological validity of neurocognitive measures in schizophrenia by quantifying aspects of subjects' ordinary activities and interactions.

**Lisa Mikesell** received her PhD in Applied Linguistics at UCLA. Her research interests include language use, social interaction, social cognition, and communication difficulties. She has used ethnographic methods and conversation analysis to better understand the needs and challenges of several populations: Generation 1.5 learners, frontotemporal dementia and schizophrenia patients, and at-risk depressed youth. She is co-author of The Interactional Instinct: The Evolution and Acquisition of Language. She is currently a postdoctoral scholar at the Semel Institute Health Services Research Center at UCLA.

**John H. Schumann** is a professor of Applied Linguistics and former chair of the Department of Applied Linguistics and TESL at UCLA. His research includes the neurobiology of language, the neurobiology of learning, language acquisition, and language evolution. He is co-author of *The Interactional Instinct: The Evolution and Acquisition of Language* (OUP, 2009) and *The Neurobiology of Language* (Erlbaum, 2004). He is also the author of *The Neurobiology of Affect in Language* (Blackwell, 1997).

**Michael Sean Smith** received his MA from and is a current doctoral student in the Department of Applied Linguistics at the University of California, Los Angeles. His research interests include talk-in-interaction, talk and the body, the ethnographic study of neurologically impaired populations, social cognition, and epistemology in mixed-method research. He has done video-recorded ethnographic work on frontotemporal dementia and is currently working on developing coding and rating measures for video-recorded data from a large observational study on individuals with schizophrenia.

**Salvatore Torrisi** is currently a doctoral candidate in the Neuroscience Inter-departmental Program at UCLA. He is researching the neural connectivity of emotion regulation in the Mood Disorders Research Program. In 2003 he received an M.F.A. in computer music composition at California Institute of the Arts and in 2007 an M.A. in Applied Linguistics at UCLA.

# —1—

# Introduction

Michael Sean Smith, Andrea W. Mates, and Lisa Mikesell

We had no idea what we were going to find, but we had to look. For years, neurologist Mario Mendez, MD, PhD and Jill Shapira, RN, PhD had been seeing frontotemporal dementia patients in their clinic, and it was becoming clear to them that the disorder's primary effect was not on cognitive function but on the patients' social function. The spouses and loved ones of these patients were bringing them in wondering if there was a reason behind a growing history of inappropriate *social* behaviors, a history that the patients themselves were not admitting to or aware of. Wanting more traction on social behaviors and social relationships, they contacted anthropologist Alan P. Fiske. Several years later, in 2005 with no funding in hand, Fiske and Mendez gathered students of social interaction and social relationships to bring multiple methods to bear on understanding social relations in frontotemporal dementia. These scholars included social psychologists, anthropologists, and applied linguists who brought together the exacting and predictive value of experimental protocols, the deep exploratory insights of ethnographic observation, and the rigid empiricism of conversation analysis. The hope was that in applying multiple methods, the different arms of the project would be able to inform and validate each other's work. In the end, there would be the documentation of social behavior in its native context, discoveries about connections between the brain and social cognition, and ultimately findings that would help patients, their families, and clinicians.

The first branch of the project to begin collecting data was the ethnography arm which followed a small number of patients in their everyday lives over a period of 6 to 24 months. The ethnographers kept records using field notes as well as video and audio tapes. The field notes allowed the ethnographers to not only record happenings but also their reactions and reflections on those happenings. The video and audio tapes provided a record that could be subject to repeated review at a later time by not only the primary ethnographer but also other members of the team. This volume is based on these kinds of data as collected by the applied linguists in the ethnography arm, a number of which are also chapter authors (A. Mates, L. Mikesell, M. Smith, and S. Torrisi).

I (A. Mates) spent most of my time with a couple we called Romeo and Juliet. Brain scans taken of Romeo nine months before I started visiting showed atrophy in frontal and inter-hemispheric regions of his brain along with an enlarged perisylvian sulcus and slightly enlarged ventricles. This along with reports from his wife and primary caregiver, Juliet, led to a diagnosis of frontotemporal dementia.

My first visit with this couple was in the evening at their Beverly Hills apartment. Driving to this unfamiliar part of town, I nervously wondered what Romeo would be like and whether all the paperwork would go smoothly. It was late fall and their living room window glowed cheerfully in the night allowing me to look in before knocking. It appeared cozy and comfortably lived in. I knocked and waited a bit before Juliet opened the door. After I entered and introduced myself, she called to the back for Romeo to come and greet me. A tall, grey-haired man with a ball cap and large glasses navigated the crowded furniture easily and gave his wife a kiss after she playfully tugged on the front of his shirt. They seemed like a sweet couple, and this helped put me at ease.

To me, Romeo could have been any quietly eccentric, older gentleman. He didn't speak to me often. He tended to be engaged in his routines and habits which mostly consisted of prayer times, preparing simple meals, and watching cable news. Being a first generation Chinese-American, I was accustomed to my elders basically ignoring me as he did. As a novice ethnographer, I didn't know to what degree research subjects might inquire about me, so I didn't think it was particularly troubling that Romeo never made such inquiries.

Juliet, on the other hand, often took breaks from her work in their home office to tell me about the latest troubling incident. Romeo might leave the water running and walk away or more frighteningly leave the stove on after making his evening popcorn. She had started to hide the potato chips he had for lunch so that he wouldn't finish the whole bag. She was experiencing a whole new relationship with him that she described as mothering. Two years earlier, she had been diagnosed with cancer, which was at that point in remission. During her treatments, he had lovingly cared for her: taking her to her appointments, helping her move around, generally attending to her every need. He had been a gregarious man with a ready laugh. He had been a man of ideas. They had moved across the country to follow dreams of becoming Hollywood screenwriters. He had had a lifelong interest in politics dating back to at least the 1968 elections. In the aftermath of the 9-11 terrorist attacks in 2001, his family members had called him from around the country asking what Al Qaeda was and what did this all mean? During a family visit back east several years later, various members had asked Juliet where did that man go? What happened to the fun, outgoing guy they were used to? Their questioning led Juliet to seek medical evaluation of his evolving condition.

The Romeo I met was a shadow of his former self. Yes, he did laugh on occasion, and he certainly watched hours of cable news, but he now had to be directed to engage in almost all activities other than getting food or going to the bathroom. When they went to church services, they no longer discussed the merits of the sermon in the car on the way home like they used to. The man who used to take it upon himself to take care of many household chores could not be relied on to water the plants without supervision. Nevertheless, he and I did develop a relationship over the two years I visited. We went on walks together, watched not only news but ballgames together, and despite dramatic decline in self-initiated activity, the last time I saw him he raised his arms for a hug while still 3 meters away from the gate. Like most relationships, there were tense times. As an observer, it was sometimes awkward to watch Juliet struggle with the many ways that the dementia disrupted their lives; and as a participant, I found myself angry with him or myself as he perseverated in certain activities. I was surprised to be so emotionally engaged in the course of conducting research. Having a background primarily in the neurobiology of language, the participant part of participant-observation ethnography was very new and at times uncomfortable. But participation in the lives of our subjects was inescapable, and the reader will find that the ethnographer authors have identified themselves openly throughout the volume. We have done so because we are interested in the social mind and the social brain, and our understanding of sociality does not come from theorizing alone, but also from our participation which has pointed us to types of interactions that warranted closer scrutiny.

## Background on Frontotemporal Dementia (FTD)

### *A brief history*

It has been over a hundred and fifteen years since the earliest cases of what we now know as frontotemporal dementia (FTD) were first described by the Prague neurologist, Arnold Pick. Though discovered almost fifteen years earlier than Alzheimer's disease, it is safe to say that much of our understanding of FTD remains incomplete. This is likely due to three factors: the fragmented study of the disease in medical history, its heterogeneous pathology, and its heterogeneous clinical presentation.

At the turn of the nineteenth century, Arnold Pick published a number of cases describing individuals who showed progressive mental deterioration typical of senile dementia but whose symptoms were limited to a specific set of abilities or behavioral disturbances (Kertesz 2004; 2007; Spatt 2003). His first documented case was of the 71 year old August H who developed an aphasic language impairment that gradually worsened over many years (Spatt 2003; Hodges 2007, 2). After August's death, Pick found in the autopsy a "pronounced atrophy of the gyri of the left hemisphere particularly on the left temporal lobe" (Kertesz 2004, 969) but no signs of focal lesions characteristic of strokes (Spatt 2003, 526). Later he examined Anna H, a 41 year old woman who showed behavioral disturbances, including decreased affect, stereotypic or repetitive behaviors, and worsening personal conduct but without any specific language impairment (Spatt 2003, 527). In that same year, Pick published his description of Anna J, a 75 year old woman who was brought into his clinic in 1900 showing abnormal behavior such as running away from her home or tearing up her garden. More interesting to Pick, however, was how her speech became increasingly "empty and repetitive," showing a "progressive loss of vocabulary" and, what he described as a "devastation of concepts" or *Verödung des Vorstellungsinhaltes* (Spatt 2003, 527). Pick's work described what we have come to know today as the three subtypes of FTD: progressive nonfluent aphasia (August H), the behavioral variant (Anna H), and semantic dementia (Anna J).

Pick himself never conducted histopathological analyses (the microscopic examination of cellular or neuronal damage) during his autopsies, instead limiting his descriptions to the macroscopic level (Karenberg 2001, 458). A histopathological description came in 1911 when Alois Alzheimer described a "circumscribed atrophy" that lacked the plaques and neurofibrils characteristic of the dementia bearing his name (Karenberg 2001, 458) but also showed intraneuronal (argyrophilic intracytoplasmic) inclusions, ballooned neurons, and "spongy cortical wasting" (Frederick 2006, 1063; Kertesz 2004, 969; Uchihara, Ikeda and Tsuchiya 2003, 321). In 1926, Onari and Spatz associated Pick's disease (PiD) with this histopathology, naming the inclusions Pick bodies, and the ballooned neurons Pick cells (Kertesz 2004, 969; Spatt 2003, 529).

Unknown at the time, the neuronal damage described by Alzheimer would only appear in a subset of patients diagnosed with Pick's. Thus using the presence of Pick bodies and other neuronal markers to diagnose Pick's disease would be unreliable especially as Pick bodies and cells were discovered in atypical cortical areas like the parietal lobes or in individuals without dementia (Uchihara *et al.* 2003, 320). This lack of correspondence finally led to the study (Constandinidis *et al.*, 1974) that confirmed that Pick's histopathology was only fully present in roughly a third of diagnosed cases. Without a clear histopathological picture or behavioral presentation, many frontal lobar cases were instead classified as non-typical Alzheimer's or simply as non-specific dementia. Subsequently, interest in these focal dementias largely disappeared in the English-speaking world over the latter half of the twentieth century (Hodges 2007, 3).

Of course, the lack of a cohesive classification did not diminish the prevalence of frontal lobe dementias, both Pick's and otherwise. In countries like Germany and Sweden, work on these dementias continued from the 1960s (Brun 2007, S3). Eventually, in the 1980s and 1990s a number of research groups from Lund, Sweden (Brun 1987; Gustafson 1987); Manchester, England (Neary *et al.* 1988); and the United States (Knopman *et al.* 1990) began reporting cases of dementia localized to the frontal and temporal lobes that showed neither the histology typical of Pick's or Alzheimer's disease, but nevertheless still had severe neuronal loss and spongiosis. Despite the lack of a consistent or even distinct histology, the continued presentation of patients with behavioral and language disturbances, as well as improvements in imaging technology, led to a renewed effort in understanding this largely marginalized dementia.

### FTD nomenclature

This rather fragmented history led to an equally fragmented nomenclature with the Lund group, the Manchester group, and the American group all establishing different terms for the same pathology. By 1994, however, the Lund and Manchester groups jointly put forward both a classification and diagnostic criteria in which frontotemporal dementia (FTD) covered frontal lobe degeneration (FLD) without Pick bodies (Kertesz 2007, S5), Pick type (PiD), and Motor Neuron Disease with Dementia (MND/D) (Amano and Iseki 1999, 418).

Oddly, this first classification did not include the language variants described by Pick. Primary progressive aphasia and semantic dementia, which were rediscovered by Marsel Mesulam in 1982 and Snowden, Goulding, and Neary in 1989 respectively, were seen as distinct from FLD pathology (Kertesz 2007, S5). This oversight was corrected in 1998 when the Lund-Manchester criteria was updated, this time using frontotemporal lobar degeneration (FTLD) to designate the whole spectrum, bvFTD for the behavioral variant, and progressive nonfluent aphasia (PNFA) and semantic dementia (SD) for the newly integrated language variants (Neary *et al.* 1998). Another group would meet later in 2000 to recommend further revisions, mostly exclusion criteria, for the Lund-Manchester (now commonly known as the Neary Criteria). Most important among the recommendations accepted was the decision to change the name for the clinical spectrum back to FTD (McKhann *et al.* 2000; Rascovsky *et al.* 2007). These transformations and revisions in nomenclature and criteria continue on, as does the push towards greater consensus on the disease. Recently, researchers have initiated an international consortium with the intent of again revising the diagnostic and research criteria for FTD, a necessity that becomes more pressing as our understanding of pharmacological and genetic therapeutic treatment grows (Rascovsky *et al.* 2007). In keeping with the current trend in terminology, we will also use FTD for the supracategory. However, because the chapter authors do not need to distinguish the behavioral variant (bvFTD) from the other variants, FTD is used to reference the behavioral variant throughout the volume, except in this introduction when specification is useful for ease of reading.

### *Epidemiology*

FTD was once thought of as a fairly rare disease (Ikeda *et al.* 2004), but is now estimated to account for 4% of all degenerative dementias (Brunnström *et al.* 2008) and 20 to 25% of early-onset dementias (Kertesz 2008, 129; Neary *et al.* 1986). In comparison to Alzheimer's disease (AD), the age of onset for FTD is earlier and the probability of developing it decreases with age. The variation in age of onset for FTD is strikingly large. In a Dutch study, although the median age of onset for FTD was 58, the ages ranged from 33 to 80 (Rosso *et al.* 2003). As for gender, it is generally considered to be 50-50, and the mean duration of the illness, from onset to death, is approximately six to eight years with a range of two to twenty (Neary *et al.* 2005; Kertesz *et al.* 2007). There seems to be a strong genetic link for FTD, though this is most relevant for the various molecular histological variants (see Kertesz 2008).

Because of the previous lack of consistency in diagnostic criteria, studies on demographics, prevalence, and incidence rates for FTD have been difficult to undertake, and of those that have been done, they are often difficult to generalize (Neary *et al.* 2005; Johnson *et al.* 2005). Although earlier studies found frequency rates as high as 28 or even 60 cases per 100,000 people per year (Constantinidis *et al.* 1985; Stevens *et al.* 1998, referenced in Ibach *et al.* 2003), recent epidemiological studies report prevalence rates ranging from 3.5 to 15.1 cases per 100,000 people (Mercy *et al.* 2008; Rosso *et al.* 2003).

Ibach *et al.* (2003, 254) suggest that the variability or under-representation of FTD may be due to several complications: diagnostic criteria may not be fully established, accepted, or practiced; FTD's overlap with psychiatric conditions; FTD's neuropathological variability; and finally the inability to count individuals suffering from FTD if they have never been forwarded to the appropriate clinic. Given these potential complications, Ibach *et al.* (2003, 261) investigated the prevalence of FTD in psychiatric institutions and found 33 individuals with FTD, 32 of whom were committed without ever being correctly diagnosed, a fact that the authors attribute to the fact that FTD often presents with behaviors similar to psychiatric disorders, affective disorders, antisocial or aggressive behavior, as well as the prevalence of alcohol abuse as an admittance reason (a common exclusion criteria for diagnostic studies). They estimate that the rate of prevalence for the general population is 48 per 100,000 for those 47 to 79 years of age and 43 per 100,000 for those 45 to 64 years of age (260).

### *The known neurobiology of FTD*

Pathologists have found that FTD patients have decreased brain weight mostly stemming from atrophy in the prefrontal and anterior temporal neocortex where the cortical laminae 1 to 3 and white matter have thinned (Chao *et al.* 2007; Brun 2007). Microscopic investigations show atrophied regions to be marked by neuronal loss, microvacuolation and astrocytic cliosis. Pick cells (ballooned neurons) are sometimes found in the temporal and frontal cortices, while  neuronal loss and gliosis have been found in the CA1 and subicular area, and ubiquinated inclusions in the dentate gyrus of the hippocampus (Graff-Radford and Woodruff 2007; Josephs 2008, 6).

The primary foci of this volume—the social, behavioral, and emotional dysfunctions associated with FTD—are typically associated with semantic dementia (SD) and the behavioral variant, bvFTD.  SD is by far the most stable in terms of localization, with atrophy primarily occurring in the anterior temporal lobes, the parahippocampal gyrus, anterior fusiform, the inferior and middle temporal gyri. Cell loss has also been observed in the ventromedial frontal cortex, posterior orbital frontal cortex, anterior cingulate, insula, amygdala, entorhinal cortex, and hippocampus (Rosen *et al.* 2002, 199). More often, however, atrophy in SD is most severe in the amygdala, anterior temporal lobes, and insular cortex, with less involvement in the cingulate or orbitofrontal cortex (Miller 2007, S20). As the atrophy, however, spreads bilaterally and affects other regions such as the ventromedial and orbitofrontal cortex or insula, one will likely see behavioral manifestations as well (Mendez *et al.* 2006; Rosen *et al.* 2002, 204).

The behavioral variant, bvFTD, shows the most variation in cortical degeneration. After the dementia has significantly progressed, the right frontal cortex may show atrophy on all sides, including the ventral, medial, and dorsolateral prefrontal cortex as well as the temporal lobes, anterior cingulate, and insula (Miller 2007, S20), though the dorsolateral area is typically spared early in the disease's progression. Early atrophy can be seen in a range of structures including the frontoinsular, the mesial frontal surface near the frontal pole, the orbitofrontal cortex, the ventromedial cortex, and anterior cingulate (Miller 2007, S20; Rosen *et al.* 2002, 204). In addition, researchers have noted both SD and bvFTD to show reduced volumes in subcortical structures such as the caudate, putamen, nucleus accumbens, with some differences in volume found in the basal ganglia (Miller 2007, S20).

Even at the macroanatomical level, the classification of FTD remains complicated with SD and bvFTD showing the most overlap but often without clear connections between localization and symptomatic presentation (Neary *et al.* 2005). SD patients will always have left temporal lobe atrophy, but not all individuals with left temporal lobe atrophy will have SD. In contrast, behavioral variant patients who have both frontal and temporal lobe atrophy may have greater atrophy in the temporal lobes but never show problems in semantic processing (Neary *et al.* 2005, 772). In addition, some patients show neuropsychological symptoms of FTD but show little to no atrophy in imaging or even at autopsy (Josephs 2008, 11). These patients can often go many years without any further behavioral deterioration (Kipps, Knibb, and Hodges 2007, 69; Kipps, Nestor, Fryer, and Hodges 2007). As a result, some researchers question whether these individuals suffer from a behavioral phenocopy or a new variant of non-progressive bv FTD (Hornberger *et al.* 2008; Hornberger *et al.* 2009). The fact that such a profusion of histopathologies and affected neuroanatomical areas can all be grouped under one condition is not a fault of indiscriminate categorization but rather due to the fact that both the language and behavioral disorders all invariably show some atrophy in either the frontal and/or temporal lobes (Neary *et al.* 2005, 771). The overlap can also be seen as a consequence of the highly interdependent processes in which ecology, language, sociality, self, and interaction find representation and are negotiated by the human brain (Seeley 2008; Seeley *et al.* 2007)

### Problems with the Diagnostic Criteria and Behavioral Profile

The revised Lund-Manchester Criteria (Neary *et al.* 1998) are still the most established diagnostic criteria for FTD (see Appendix A). Change in social behavior is by far the most predominate feature of FTD distinguishing it from AD, and is often defined by the presence of impaired social interaction (Kipps *et al.* 2009, 593; Neary *et al.* 2005, 774). Patients are often seen as lacking social emotions like sympathy, empathy, shame, or guilt. They may also develop stereotyped behaviors from simple physical and verbal repetitions to complex routines, as well as alterations in eating habits such as gluttony or preference for sweets (Neary *et al.* 2005, 774). There seems to be few "phenotypic variations" in which patients either become indifferent, disinhibited, hyperactive, and gregarious, or conversely, grow apathetic, abulic (lacking initiative), and emotionally blunted (Neary *et al.* 2005, 774). Recent functional imaging studies and autopsy studies suggest that the disinhibited phenotype involves orbitofrontal and anterior temporal lobes, while the apathetic phenotype regularly involves extensive frontal involvement including the dorsolateral prefrontal cortex (Neary *et al.* 2005, 774). Greater involvement in the right frontal cortex usually predicts greater abnormal social behavior (Neary *et al.* 2005, 774).

Issues of identification and diagnosis of FTD have always been at the forefront of clinical research and practice. An ongoing concern for clinicians is that, because of the lack of public knowledge about FTD and the fact that it results in behavioral (as opposed to cognitive) impairment, many individuals suffering from FTD are often misdiagnosed or sometimes not even suspected of having dementia (Graham 2007, 29). This is complicated by the fact that most clinical tasks are cognitive assessments. As such, neuropsychological performance for bvFTD patients may remain normal for an extended period of time despite the disease's progression (Kipps *et al.* 2009). Another complication in the diagnostic process is patients' lack of insight (i.e., unawareness of their behavioral changes) and lack of concern for others. Because of this ignorance, patients rarely self-refer to a physician. This is in contrast to other dementias like Alzheimer's, Parkinson's, or the aphasic variant, PNFA, where the individual is as likely to seek medical help as his or her family (Pijnenburg *et al.* 2004). For instance, one study (Chow *et al.* 2005) found that while aphasic or memory patients often self-referred directly to specialty clinics, bvFTD patients were often presented first to general clinics by others and also had a lower representation at specialty clinics. In clinic, they were often misadiagnosed because of the primarily behavioral, as opposed to cognitive, presentation of bvFTD. Diagnoses of bvFTD patients are delayed by a mean of two years, and are given diagnoses like memory disorder, mood disorder, hypochondrias, cerebrovascular disease, or no diagnosis at all. This is in contrast to primary progressive aphasia, which was rarely misdiagnosed (Pijnenburg *et al.* 2004).

The difficulty in diagnosis is often attributed to the complexity and variability of core and supporting features (McKhann *et al.* 2001). Only a minority of patients show all the core features at presentation while certain supportive features like stereotypy or compulsive behaviors are often common in early stages (Mendez and Perryman 2002, 425–426). Furthermore, some clinicians argue that the diagnostic criteria are "...subjective, and lack reliable scales to guide the user on items such as "emotional blunting" or "regulation of personal conduct"" and become problematic for inter-rater reliability among clinical workers, especially when greater inference into the patient's cognitive or emotional state is required (Rascovsky *et al.* 2007, S15–16). As a result of these difficulties with the current diagnostic tools, many researchers have been moving towards incorporating assessments from other disciplines including theory of mind (ToM) tasks or measures of social cognition from developmental psychology (Kipps and Hodges 2006; Torralva *et al.* 2007. Interestingly, some clinicians have shown promising results assessing "acquired sociopathy" in FTD patients by relying less on cognitive tasks and more on behavioral measures originally developed for forensic psychologists (Mendez, Chen, Shapira, and Miller 2005; Rankin *et al.* 2008).

### Caregivers and clinical care

The difficulty in identifying individuals with FTD begins long before an individual is brought to a physician. Like other dementias, FTD follows a course that is gradual, that is, the affected areas of the brain slowly atrophy, causing some delay between the physical onset of the disease and its observable effects on the individual. FTD's onset, however, is also described as *insidious*. As such, caregivers do not often suspect a mental illness until the patient's disturbances become so noticeable that they are no longer able to be ignored or explained. Following diagnosis, caregivers often retrospectively interpret early and often subtle changes in the individual as attributable to the disease.

The slow distortion in the individual's character and social conduct is captured in the Neary criteria (Neary *et al.* 1998, see Appendix A) as "early decline in social interpersonal and personal conduct," "loss of sympathy or empathy," "disinhibited speech and gestures, and violations of interpersonal space," and "loss of emotional warmth, empathy, and sympathy, and indifference to others." These features, however, also co-occur with the individual's growing *lack of insight* into his or her changing behavior or others' reactions to those changes. There is little certainty in how the changes begin, as opposed to when they are noticed by others, and whether these changes start as simple exaggerations in the person's prior personality or as mild eccentricities (Kipps, Knibb and Hodges 2007, 42, 47). Even when the individual's behaviors become radically different, and others become concerned, this does not always guarantee that dementia will be a suspected cause. Often, others will either attribute the behavior, such as apathy or depression, to more benign problems, (Kipps, Knibb and Hodges 2007, 43), or they may make attributions about the individual, which may be innocuous or more condemning of the individual's character or moral failings. Even after diagnosis caregivers often become hurt and angered by the patients because they have trouble treating the patient's behaviors or lack of concern as symptoms of the disease (Lough and Garfoot 2007, 302). It is not surprising then that prior to diagnosis and without an alternative account for the individual's behavior, these changes would erode the individual's relationships to the point of estrangement, divorce, or abandonment long before he or she is brought in for medical attention. This is again suggested by the Ibach *et al.* (2003) study. Of the 33 institutionalized FTD patients, only one had previously been diagnosed. Another report details a lieutenant colonel in the United States Air Force, whom, over a nine year progression of the illness, was investigated for downloading pornography onto a government computer, attacked his young nephew at a family wedding, left for two years of active service in South Korea without telling his family, and was subsequently demoted and discharged from the military, divorced by his wife, and alienated from his family. He was finally taken to the emergency room by his sister after seeing his living conditions, but not before he urinated on his living room floor and defecated in her car (Faber *et al.* 2003).

The long road from behavioral change to diagnosis, with all its potential pitfalls, puts tremendous strain on the people close to the person suffering from FTD. FTD affects more than just the individual, but also the social networks in which the individual participates, whether that be family, friendships, or community. One study looking at the psychosocial consequences of bvFTD (Passant *et al.* 2005) found many dramatic changes: "teetotalers" beginning to abuse alcohol (S16), some patients becoming verbally abusive in public, others losing social propriety and urinating in public or getting into traffic accidents without concern, shoplifting, giving away large amounts of money to strangers, and other odd or aberrant behaviors. One patient even set fire to his bed. Given that patients lack insight into their disease and concern about their behaviors, caregivers and family members may be the ones who truly suffer on account of the dementia.

The orientation of clinical work in FTD can also be said to be a product of and sensitive to the disease's impact on others. This is seen in its treatment, which can be characterized as psychosocial with a greater emphasis on the family as the entity being treated rather than the individual alone (Lough and Garfoot 2007). Caregivers are also important to the diagnostic process, providing clinicians with essential information about the patient's behavioral changes. In fact, clinicians rely on informant reports in assessing the patient when determining diagnosis even more than neuropsychological or imaging abnormalities (Kipps *et al.* 2009), which are used as corroborative measures only (Mendez, McMurtray, Chen, Shapira, Mishkin and Miller 2005, 4). Clinics often use informant rating scales including the Cambridge Behavioural Inventory (CBI; Bozeat *et al.* 2000), the Neuropsychiatric Inventory (NPI; Cummings *et al.* 1994), the Frontal Behavioral Inventory (FBI; Kertesz *et al.* 2003a), and the Frontal Behavioral Score (FBS; Lebert *et al.* 1998) (all referenced in Kipps, Knibb and Hodges 2007, 46), which ask caregivers to assess the patient's behaviors as compared to the patient's prior behaviors (e.g., prefers sweet foods more than before; shows less enthusiasm for his/her usual interests, CBI; Bozeat *et al.* 2000), or as problematic in comparison to an implied norm of conduct (e.g., is uncooperative when asked to do something; talks to total strangers as if they know them, CBI; Bozeat *et al.* 2000). While these scales often have good retest and inter-rater reliability, there is often a concern that informants are relied on too much and instead there is a need for behavioral or cognitive evaluations that can assess FTD by examining the patient him or herself (Lough and Garfoot 2007, 281). The reliance on informants demonstrates how other's evaluations of FTD patients' behavior as socially appropriate or inappropriate become a constitutive feature of the pathology.

## Significance of this Volume

The description of FTD as a pathological change in social behavior provides the motivation for applying ethnographic and interactional approaches to FTD in natural social contexts. We argue that these approaches do more than document the disease and its effects on family, friends, and colleagues by revealing phenomena that can be analyzed empirically as causing systematic changes in the patient's social interactions. The insidious onset of the disease and how others come to interpret changes in the individual's conduct and personality suggest that the deterioration in the individual shows a transformation that is still interpretable by others, even if negatively, as an interactional process. This not only suggests a transformation in the patient's sociality, but more importantly, suggests a transformation that is often, for others, inescapably moral in nature. The current need for informants in clinical diagnosis and the successful use of evaluative rather than descriptive features, however, also suggest that the particular behaviors displayed are less significant than the conflict these behaviors cause in social contexts. Study of how others come to define the patients' actions in situated contexts provides a perspective on FTD as an interactional product that is detectable in clinical research, but not fully observable. The same could be proposed of research exploring how FTD affects emotional expression or motivation in engagement with others. Since FTD's rediscovery in recent decades, interest has grown not only with respect to the problems it presents for clinical diagnosis or behavioral description, but also with respect to how those problems provide a unique window into how the brain produces language, organizes meaning, and carries out social and moral reasoning. Conversely, FTD has also shown us how important social and interactional processes are for our understanding of the human brain, and how much our lack of understanding of these processes impoverishes our understanding of this dementia. Social science methods, especially ethnographic or interactional, are then in a unique position to contribute to our understanding of FTD, and how the brain and interaction produces the social mind.

As noted earlier, this volume is the result of a serendipitous meeting between researchers at the Focal-Type Dementia Clinic and researchers in the Department of Anthropology at UCLA, which has since blossomed into an ongoing multi-disciplinary research group led by Dr. Mario Mendez and Dr. Alan P. Fiske. This research project brings together multiple methods and perspectives and this volume reports on some of the findings stemming from the deep exploratory insights of ethnographic observation and the rigid empiricism of conversation analysis (CA) (see Fiske, Chapter 8, this volume for more on this unique collaboration). Through actual documentation of social behavior in action, this project hopes to eventually provide better tools for diagnosis and resources for caregiver counseling as well as provide greater insight into the connections between the brain and social cognition.

We take seriously the title of the work, the "reverse engineering of the social mind," and hope in the end the reader does as well. Reverse engineering is a process in which engineers take a finished product and study its internal mechanisms and external output post hoc. The goal of reverse engineering may be to understand the product's inner workings well enough to simply describe them to others, to modify the product, or to create a similar product. Our approach to research into social interaction is also to emphasize the "final product"—actual behaviors—and how people actually interact while using the brains they have that day at that moment. In this pursuit, we feel that we are taking up the challenge set forth by Marsel Mesulam in his contribution to *The Principles of Frontal Lobe Functioning*:

> [T]he mechanisms that shape the course of individual actions are currently beyond the scope of neurological analysis. Perhaps this will become possible when a new science is developed for analyzing not only how a single brain reacts to experience but also how brains (and their owners) interact with each other to form social matrices, which then influence individual decisions. (Mesulam 2002, 26)

We take then social interaction, as the beginning and core of our analyses. As a consequence, it is important to distinguish the conclusions reached in the chapters herein from the analyses of the particular interactional excerpts. Our methodological purpose is to "discover" or observe frontotemporal dementia as a social pathology being produced by the interaction between the patients' actions, the events and actions of others occurring around them, and how this constitutes the pathology of the individual in the social experience of others. We wish to reveal frontotemporal dementia as observable phenomena, as it manifests in the context that it first appeared—in interaction with others—and show it in such a way that anyone, whether clinician, psychologist, or social scientist, can also look at the data, see the same phenomena, and evaluate the basis for the claims made. Even if the conclusions reached are eventually countered or modified, the utterly empirical nature of this research, its subject, and what it can provide for those interested in the brain, mental illness, language, and social interaction, is a powerful and unique contribution that this work makes. If we have accomplished our most simple objective—to show and describe the events and actions occurring in the data in accordance with how the actual interactants treated them—we have presented a description of reality that embeds a clinico-pathology in social interaction, the primordial site that the *homo sapien* brain has evolved in and evolved for and to which all theories of social functioning whether neurological, psychological, or linguistic must ultimately be held accountable.

Given the aims of this volume, most chapters approach FTD from an ethnomethodological perspective. They employ ethnographic methods and/ or CA to explore various issues related to FTD and social functioning. Chapter 2 uses these methods to better understand the brain regions that subserve social functioning. In this chapter, Torrisi demonstrates the usefulness of combining methodologies to examine the inappropriate social behaviors of FTD and better understand the brain areas underlying such behaviors. He presents a case study of an FTD patient and details her behaviors using ethnographic data and video recordings of her interactions in ordinary social contexts. He then discusses this patient's brain imaging results, showing how understanding the functions of the affected regions helps explain her inappropriate social behaviors.

Chapters 3 through 5 use CA to provide a detailed and rigorously empirical description of FTD patients' behaviors and discuss the ways in which caregivers respond to such behaviors. These three chapters illustrate how examining natural interactions of FTD patients can have clinical relevance. In Chapter 3, Smith analyzes the moral structure of interactions between FTD patients and their interlocutors, arguing that while issues of transgression and violation are central to the social presentation of FTD, their underlying bases may rest on simpler social processes like insensibility and incongruity. He further shows how the difficulty patients and their co-participants experience in interaction may be predicated on how fitted the current course of action is to the patient's person-specific interests or self-same concept. In Chapter 4, Mikesell examines the perseverative behaviors of an FTD patient showing how these behaviors disrupt the social order of interaction. She finds that interlocutors use three practices to manage this patient's perseverative behaviors with each practice having differing effects on the ongoing interaction. She discusses the clinical relevance of this work as well as the how this work contributes to an understanding of normal social functioning and caregiver stress. Avineri, in Chapter 5, uses CA to examine FTD interactions in the clinic. Specifically, she investigates how FTD patients, who are described as lacking insight, display insight and how other interlocutors including clinicians orient to insight during clinical interviews. She claims that insight is a multifaceted concept that surfaces through interactional collaboration.

Chapters 6 through 9 are extensions of the ethnomethodological approaches employed throughout the book. These chapters incorporate what has been learned from ethnomethodological studies of FTD interactions in order to consider a possible neurobiology of a common discourse practice, that of person reference (Chapter 6), to show the involvement of the prefrontal cortices in the process of socialization and loss of the ability to implement what has been learned during the process of socialization (Chapter 7), to investigate the role of social motives and moral emotions in sustaining relationships (Chapter 8), and to reflect on the state of the field of applied linguistics (Chapter 9). In Chapter 6, Mates proposes a neurobiological substrate of a discourse practice, that of person reference. Examining natural interaction, she presents several cases in which FTD patients inappropriately under- or over-suppose their interlocutor's knowledge about the persons they are referring to in photographs, which is notably different from normals' person reference practices during a similar task. Based on this finding, she argues that FTD patients' atrophy of particular brain regions is likely responsible for this deficit. She then argues for probable brain areas underlying person reference, a well-studied and common discourse practice in ordinary conversation. In Chapter 7, Joaquin uses ethnographic data to compare two populations: children with under-developed prefrontal cortices and FTD patients with degenerating prefrontal cortices (PFC). In doing so, she shows that both populations often display social "deficits" or socially inappropriate behaviors and are often sanctioned by caregivers in similar ways. Combining this evidence with a review of the literature on the functions of the prefrontal cortices, she argues that the PFC is essential for learning and implementing social norms. In Chapter 8, Fiske argues that FTD patients' inappropriate behaviors are caused by a loss of social motives and moral emotions. Fiske incorporates data collected in ethnomethodological traditions to characterize the nature of such losses and to illustrate their impact on relationships. Although patients retain that ability to reason, Fiske argues that it is this loss of social motives and moral emotions that drastically affects the quality of patients' relationships, leading Fiske to deduce that rational behavior alone cannot sustain satisfying relationships. Schumann, in Chapter 9, reflects on what the study of FTD patients' social interactions has contributed to the field of applied linguistics. He extends past work on the role of the prefrontal cortex in language pragmatics and argues that FTD-caregiver interactions are an example of how culture and society can act as an external prefrontal cortex modulating behavior.

Taken together, all of the chapters in this volume demonstrate how studies of the social interactions and discourse practices of FTD patients and their interlocutors can contribute to a more accurate and precise description of FTD behaviors, to a more sympathetic understanding of caregiver challenges, to an awareness of the typical expectations of social appropriateness, and to an understanding of normal social functioning, the maintenance of relationships, and language pragmatics. Additionally, many of the chapters illustrate how such studies can have clinical implications, show the importance of contextualizing patients' behaviors, and demonstrate how caregivers' management practices require a distributed and coordinated effort. Lastly, we hope that all the chapters encourage curiosity and pursuance of difficult issues by presenting a unique forum for considering interdisciplinary questions that may not, at least at this time, have obvious answers.

## References


Amano, N. and E. Iseki.

1999 Introduction: Pick's disease and frontotemporal dementia. *Neuropathology* 19(4): 417–421.

Bozeat, S., C.A. Gregory, M.A.L. Ralph and J.R. Hodges.

2000 Which neuropsychiatric and behavioural features distinguish frontal and temporal variants of frontotemporal dementia from Alzheimer's disease? *Journal of Neurology, Neurosurgery, and Psychiatry*, 69(2): 178–186.

Brun, A.

1987 Frontal lobe degeneration of non-Alzheimer type. I. Neuropathology. *Archives of Gerontology and Geriatrics* 6(3): 193–208.

2007 Identification and characterization of frontal lobe degeneration: historical perspective on the development of FTD. *Alzheimer Disease and Associated Disorders* 21(4): S3–4.

Brunnström, H., L. Gustafson, U. Passant and E. Englund.

2008 Prevalence of dementia subtypes: A 30-year retrospective survey of neuropathological reports. *Archives of Gerontology and Geriatrics*. doi: 10.1016/j. archger.2008.06.005

Chao, L.L., N. Schuff, E.M. Clevenger, S.G. Mueller, H.J. Rosen, M.L. Gorno-Tempini, J.H. Kramer; B.L. Miller and M.W. Weiner.

2007  Patterns of White Matter Atrophy in Frontotemporal Lobar Degeneration. *Archives of Neurology* 64(11): 1619

Chow, T.W., J.R. Hodges, K.E. Dawson, B.L. Miller, V. Smith, M.F. Mendez and A.M. Lipton.

2005  Referral Patterns for Syndromes Associated With Frontotemporal Lobar Degeneration. *Alzheimer disease and associated disorders* 19(1): 17–19

Constantinidis, J., J. Richard, and R. Tissot

1974  Pick's disease: Histological and clinical correlations. *European Neurology* 11: 208–217.

1985  Pick dementia: Anatomoclinical correlations and pathophysiological considerations. *Interdisciplinary Topics in Gerontolology* 19: 72–97.

Cummings, J.L., M. Mega, K. Gray, S. Rosenberg-Thompson, D.A. Carusi and J. Gornbein.

1994  The Neuropsychiatric Inventory: comprehensive assessment of psychopathology in dementia. *Neurology* 44(12): 2308–2314.

Faber, R., V.M. Hill and B.J. Kim.

2003  Frontotemporal dementia affecting a U.S. Air Force officer. *Military Medicine* 168(4): 333–336.

Frederick, J.

2006  Pick disease: a brief overview. *Archives of Pathology and Laboratory Medicine* 130(7): 1063–1066.

Graff-Radford, N.R. and B.K. Woodruff.

2007  Frontotemporal Dementia. *Seminars in Neurology* 27(1): 48–57.

Graham, A.

2007  *Epidemiology of frontotemporal dementia. In Frontotemporal dementia syndromes*, edited by J.R. Hodges, 25–37. Cambridge: Cambridge University Press.

Gustafson, L.

1987  Frontal lobe degeneration of non-Alzheimer type. II. Clinical picture and differential diagnosis. *Archives of Gerontology and Geriatrics* 6(3): 209–223.

Hodges, J.R.

2007  Overview of Frontotemporal Dementia. In *Frontotemporal Dementia Syndromes,* edited by J.R. Hodges, 1–24. Cambridge: Cambridge University Press.

Hornberger, M., O. Piguet, C. Kipps and J.R. Hodges.

2008  Executive function in progressive and nonprogressive behavioral variant frontotemporal dementia. *Neurology* 71(19): 1481–1488.

Hornberger, M., B.P. Shelley, C.M. Kipps, O. Piguet and J.R. Hodges.

2009  Can progressive and non-progressive behavioral variant frontotemporal dementia be distinguished at presentation? *Journal of Neurology, Neurosurgery, and Psychiatry*. doi: 10.1136/jnnp.2008.163873.

Ibach, B., H. Koch, M. Koller and M. Wolfersdorf.

2003  Hospital admission circumstances and prevalence of frontotemporal lobar degeneration: a multicenter psychiatric state hospital study in Germany. *Dementia and Geriatric Cognitive Disorders* 16(4): 253–264.

Ikeda, M., T. Ishikawa and H. Tanabe.

2004  Epidemiology of frontotemporal lobar degeneration. *Dementia and Geriatric Cognitive Disorders* 17(4): 265–268.

Johnson, J.K., J. Diehl, M.F. Mendez, J. Neuhaus, J.S. Shapira, M. Forman, D.J. Chute, E.D. Roberson, C. Pace-Savitsky, M. Neumann, T.W. Chow, H.J. Rosen, H. Forstl, A. Kurz and B.L. Miller.

2005  Frontotemporal lobar degeneration: demographic characteristics of 353 patients. *Archives of Neurology* 62(6): 925–930.

Josephs, K.A.

2008  Frontotemporal dementia and related disorders: deciphering the enigma. *Annals of Neurology* 64(1): 4–14.

Karenberg, A.

2001  [Early history of Pick's disease]. *Fortschritte Der Neurologie-Psychiatrie* 69(11): 545–550

Kertesz, A., W. Davidson, P. McCabe and D. Munoz.

2003  Behavioral quantitation is more sensitive than cognitive testing in frontotemporal dementia. *Alzheimer Disease and Associated Disorders* 17(4): 223–229.

Kertesz, A.

2004  Frontotemporal Dementia/Pick's Disease. *Archives of Neurology* 61(6): 969–971.

2007  Pick complex--historical introduction. *Alzheimer Disease and Associated Disorders* 21(4): S5–7.

2008  Frontotemporal dementia: a topical review. *Cognitive and Behavioral Neurology: Official Journal of the Society for Behavioral and Cognitive Neurology,*

21(3): 127–133.

Kertesz, A., M. Blair, P. McMonagle and D.G. Munoz.

2007 The diagnosis and course of frontotemporal dementia. *Alzheimer Disease and Associated Disorders* 21(2): 155–163.

Kipps, C.M. and J.R. Hodges.

2006 Theory of mind in frontotemporal dementia. *Social Neuroscience* 1(3): 235–244.

Kipps, C.M., P.J. Nestor, J. Acosta-Cabronero, R. Arnold and J.R. Hodges.

2009 Understanding social dysfunction in the behavioural variant of frontotemporal dementia: the role of emotion and sarcasm processing. *Brain: A Journal of Neurology.*

Kipps, C.M., P.J. Nestor, T.D. Fryer and J.R. Hodges.

2007 Behavioural variant frontotemporal dementia: not all it seems? *Neurocase: Case Studies in Neuropsychology, Neuropsychiatry, and Behavioural Neurology* 13(4): 237–247.

Kipps, C., J. Knibb and J.R. Hodges.

2007 Clinical presentations of frontotemporal dementia. In *Frontotemporal Dementia Syndromes*, edited by J.R. Hodges, 38–79. Cambridge University Press.

Knopman, D.S., A.R. Mastri, W.H. Frey, J.H. Sung and T. Rustan.

1990 Dementia lacking distinctive histologic features: a common non-Alzheimer degenerative dementia. *Neurology* 40(2): 251–256.

Lebert, F., F. Pasquier, L. Souliez and H. Petit.

1998 Frontotemporal behavioral scale. *Alzheimer Disease and Associated Disorders.* 12(4): 335–339.

Lough, S. and V. Garfoot.

2007 Psychological interventions in frontotemporal dementia. In *Frontotemporal Dementia Syndromes*, edited by J.R. Hodges, 277–325. Cambridge: Cambridge University Press.

McKhann, G.M., M.S. Albert, M. Grossman, B. Miller, D. Dickson and J.Q. Trojanowski.

2001 Clinical and pathological diagnosis of frontotemporal dementia: report of the Work Group on Frontotemporal Dementia and Pick's Disease. *Archives of Neurology* 58(11): 1803–1809.

Mendez, M.F., A.K. Chen, J.S. Shapira, P. Lu and B.L. Miller.

2006 Acquired extroversion associated with bitemporal variant of frontotemporal dementia. *The Journal of Neuropsychiatry and Clinical Neurosciences.* 18(1): 100–107.

Mendez, M.F., A.K. Chen, J.S. Shapira and B.L. Miller.
2005  Acquired sociopathy and frontotemporal dementia. *Dementia and Geriatric Cognitive Disorders* 20(2–3): 99–104.

Mendez, M.F., A. McMurtray, A.K. Chen, J.S. Shapira, F. Mishkin and B.L. Miller.
2005  Functional neuroimaging and presenting psychiatric features in frontotemporal dementia. *Journal of Neurology, Neurosurgery, and Psychiatry* 77: 4–7.

Mendez, M.F. and K.M. Perryman.
2002  Neuropsychiatric Features of Frontotemporal Dementia: Evaluation of Consensus Criteria and Review. *J Neuropsychiatry Clin Neurosci* 14(4): 424–429.

Mercy, L., J.R. Hodges, K. Dawson, R.A. Barker and C. Brayne.
2008  Incidence of early-onset dementias in Cambridgeshire, United Kingdom. *Neurology* 71(19): 1496–1499.

Mesulam, M.
2002  The Human Frontal Lobes: Transcending the Default Mode through Contingent Encoding. In *Principles of frontal lobe function,* edited by D.T. Stuss and R.T. Knight, 8–30. Oxford: Oxford University Press.

Miller, B.L.
2007  Frontotemporal dementia and semantic dementia: anatomic variations on the same disease or distinctive entities? *Alzheimer Disease and Associated Disorders* 21(4): S19–22.

Neary, D., J.S. Snowden, B. Northen and P. Goulding.
1988  Dementia of frontal lobe type. *Journal of Neurology, Neurosurgery, and Psychiatry* 51(3): 353–361.

Neary, D., J.S. Snowden, D.M. Bowen, N.R. Sims, D.M. Mann, J.S. Benton, B. Northen, P.O. Yates and A.N. Davison.
1986  Neuropsychological syndromes in presenile dementia due to cerebral atrophy. *Journal of Neurology, Neurosurgery, and Psychiatry* 49(2): 163–174.

Neary, D., J.S. Snowden, L. Gustafson, U. Passant, D. Stuss, S. Black, M. Freedman, A. Kertesz, P.H. Robert, M. Albert, K. Boone, B.L. Miller, J. Cummings and D.F. Benson.
1998  Frontotemporal lobar degeneration: A consensus on clinical diagnostic criteria. *Neurology* 51(6): 1546–1554.

Neary, D., J. Snowden and D. Mann.

2005 Frontotemporal dementia. *The Lancet Neurology* 4(11): 771–780.

Passant, U., C. Elfgren, E. Englund, and L. Gustafson

2005 Psychiatric symptoms and their psychosocial consequences in frontotemporal dementia. *Alzheimer Disease and Associated Disorders* 19: S15–S18.

Pijnenburg, Y.A.L., F. Gillissen, C. Jonker and P. Scheltens.

2004 Initial complaints in frontotemporal lobar degeneration. *Dementia and Geriatric Cognitive Disorders* 17(4): 302–306.

Rankin, K.P., W. Santos-Modesitt, J.H. Kramer, D. Pavlic, V. Beckman and B.L. Miller.

2008 Spontaneous social behaviors discriminate behavioral dementias from psychiatric disorders and other dementias. *The Journal of Clinical Psychiatry* 69(1): 60–73.

Rascovsky, K., J.R. Hodges, C.M. Kipps, J.K. Johnson, W.W. Seeley, M.F. Mendez, et al.

2007 Diagnostic criteria for the behavioral variant of frontotemporal dementia (bvFTD): current limitations and future directions. *Alzheimer Disease and Associated Disorders* 21(4): S14–18.

Rosen, H.J., M.L. Gorno-Tempini, W.P. Goldman, R.J. Perry, N. Schuff, M. Weiner, R. Feiwell, J.H. Kramer and B.L. Miller.

2002 Patterns of brain atrophy in frontotemporal dementia and semantic dementia. *Neurology.* 58(2): 198–208.

Rosso, S.M., L. Donker Kaat, T. Baks, M. Joosse, I. de Koning, Y. Pijnenburg, D. de Jong, D. Dooijes, W. Kamphorst, R. Ravid, M.F. Niermeijer, F. Verheij, H.P. Kremer, P. Scheltens, C.M. van Duijn, P. Heutink and J.C. van Swieten.

2003 Frontotemporal dementia in The Netherlands: patient characteristics and prevalence estimates from a population-based study. *Brain: A Journal of Neurology.* 126(Pt 9): 2016–2022.

Seeley, W.W.

2008 Selective functional, regional, and neuronal vulnerability in frontotemporal dementia. *Current Opinion in Neurology.* 21(6): 701–707.

Seeley, W.W., J.M. Allman, D.A. Carlin, R.K. Crawford, M.N. Macedo, M.D. Greicius, S.J. DeArmond and B.L. Miller.

2007 Divergent social functioning in behavioral variant frontotemporal dementia and Alzheimer disease: reciprocal networks and neuronal evolution. *Alzheimer Disease and Associated Disorders.* 21(4): S50–57.

Spatt, Josef.

2003. Arnold Pick's concept of dementia. *Cortex* 39 (3): 525-531.

Stevens, M., C.M. van Duijn, W. Kamphorst, P. de Knijff, P. Heutink, W.A. van Gool, P. Scheltens, R. Ravid, B.A. Oostra, M.F. Niermeijer and J.C. van Swieten.

1998 Familial aggregation in frontotemporal dementia. *Neurology.* 50(6): 1541–1545.

Torralva, T., C.M. Kipps, J.R. Hodges, L. Clark, T. Bekinschtein, M. Roca, María Lujan Calcagno and Facundo Manes.

2007 The relationship between affective decision-making and theory of mind in the frontal variant of fronto-temporal dementia. *Neuropsychologia.* 45(2): 342–349.

Uchihara, T., K. Ikeda and K. Tsuchiya.

2003 Pick body disease and Pick syndrome.* *Neuropathology.* 23(4): 318–326.

# — 2 —

# Social Regulation in Frontotemporal Dementia: A Case Study

Salvatore Torrisi

## Overview and Introduction

People regulate their actions in social contexts. A typical interaction between two individuals may require such disparate regulatory skills as deciding when or how to phrase an utterance, whether or not to delay or stifle an inappropriate impulse, or modify a behavior to match what is prosocial and helpful for another. As psychologist Jennifer Beer writes, "social regulation occurs when people exert control over their interpersonal behavior to match their internal standards and expectations, instead of merely reacting to properties of environmental stimuli" (Beer 2006, 154).

In this chapter, social regulation is construed not as a single psychological construct but involves a number of different cognitive and emotional processes (Baumeister and Heatherton 1996; Beer and Ochsner 2006; Gross 2001; Lieberman and Pfeifer 2005). Some of these processes are predicated on the perception and monitoring of one's *self*. Other processes are predicated on the *other* individual in a social dyad, such as considering or imagining what the other knows or may be thinking. Such processes are often referred to as having "theory of mind" (Premack and Woodruff 1978). And still other processes are predicated on socially-relevant *emotions* that arise when interacting with others. All these processes can be thought to exist against a backdrop of learned declarative knowledge and cultural rules for what one should or should not do in a social context.

Despite the rather broad nature of this construct (which later sections shall flesh out further), it is clear to effectively regulate social behavior one needs: a) social standards by which to evaluate ongoing or potential actions, b) an awareness of self, c) awareness of an other, d) the experience of an emotion, no matter how subtle, that arises during interactions, and e) regulatory mechanisms that control and direct one's behaviors accordingly. Breakdown at any one of these levels can result in abnormal social behaviors. Social neuroscience is currently revealing the neurobiological basis of many of the psychological requirements for social regulation, and despite advances in modern imaging technologies, the traditional neurological study of individuals with brain abnormalities is still very useful to this research. This is because damage to or the absence of particular anatomical areas can reveal the functional contributions they make to larger networks.

It is important, however, to remember that psychological functions are heterogeneously localized and that their anatomical localization is generally distributed across the brain; therefore the resulting cognitive and behavioral profiles of brain damaged persons cannot always be easily attributed to simple region-function mappings. Because virtually every brain region serves multiple functions, especially outside primary sensory cortex, and serves some functions more effectively than others, damage to one or more regions creates a "matrix" of syndromes (Damasio 1994, 56).

Despite repudiating this simple cognitive modularity, connections between structure and function can still be drawn with some level of confidence. Neurologists, and more recently neuroscientists and psychologists, have come to observe that a particular kind of focal pathology and the abnormal behaviors that stem from it can illuminate the networks that particularly serve social cognition. A careful look at an individual with such a neuropathology, frontotemporal dementia (see Chapter 1 for introduction), may contribute something to our understanding of social regulation in the brain.

## Kelly

Kelly, age 52, earned a Ph.D. in piano performance from a prestigious university. She made her living giving private lessons and judging piano competitions. She was described by her husband, Bron, as once a very warm and approachable person as well as a born teacher with an uncanny ability to communicate with her students. Throughout the school year she would buy things that reminded her of particular students to give to them as prizes during annual recitals and picnics she organized. She was also a valued professional among her colleagues and was on track to become president of a musical association to which she belonged. Kelly made friends easily, was rarely disliked, and on the rare occasions when criticism came her way she was very sensitive to it. Always polite, she did not like confrontation and would rarely press her point of view or request her desires too boldly.

Around 2003, Kelly began to exhibit gradual changes in these characteristics. Understandably, this period was one of great pain and confusion for Bron. Since 2004 he has seen a rapid increase in the rate of Kelly's cognitive and emotional decline. She became too difficult for Bron to manage alone so he sought outside care. While able for some time to find sanctuary in a care facility, Kelly became so socially disruptive, aggressive and difficult to manage that she was expelled. At the time of this study Kelly had been successfully relocated with an increased dosage of certain medications.

In late 2005, Kelly underwent her first neurological assessment. As typical for a neurological consultation, her illness history was reviewed, her caregiver (Bron) was interviewed, she was given a number of physical and neuropsychological tests, structural MRI and functional PET scans were obtained and a diagnosis was made with a prognosis for treatment and therapy. At the time, the primary description of "semantic dementia" was given, qualified with "...other manifestations of a frontotemporal lobar degeneration[1]... including personality changes with some dysexecutive functioning, detachment, disinhibition, decreased emotional processing, and decreased insight" (UCLA FTD and Neurobehavior Clinic 2005, 2006). The following year Kelly's diagnosis shifted emphasis and was described as semantic dementia "...evolving more into the associated socioemotional and other behavioral changes consistent with this syndrome." Kelly presents with a "mix" of cognitive and emotional deficits. A number of these cognitive deficits are quite glaring.

First, Kelly perseverates with complex compulsive behaviors. These stereotyped and perseverative behaviors are quite complicated, involving multiple stages and a substantial amount of time to complete. She has gone through a number of different fixations on which she perseverates, and one which has proved both frequent and enduring is to ask what time it is to check her medication schedule (see Mikesell, Chapter 4 for analysis). Interestingly, clock-watching and schedule-checking have been frequently reported in semantic dementia and/or the temporal lobe variant of FTD (Rosso *et al.* 2001; Snowden *et al.* 1996, 101).

Second, Kelly has a severe impairment in her recognition of word meaning. This is a curious type of language dysfunction, where it is the concept of the word or object that deteriorates, rather than, for example, the ability to pronounce it. On the mini Boston Naming Test (Kaplan *et al.* 1983), a neuropsychological assessment of object recognition, Kelly correctly identified only

---

1.    This is a common clinical superordinate category for FTD, which also includes primary progressive aphasia and semantic dementia.

2 out of 15 items. On a different task, she was asked to describe particular objects. She defined a carrot as a fruit, green, and sweet. She also had trouble recognizing words such as kettle and ladle.

Third, Kelly has experienced a severe breakdown in her ability to process and identify faces, clinically called prosopagnosia. On a test of twenty photos of famous faces, she could not identify any. This breakdown was not only limited to famous faces but also close individuals. On a joint visit to the care facility, Bron had to inform Kelly that the man she had just walked by without recognizing was her own brother.

Thus far, Kelly's cognitive, as opposed to emotional, deficits have been described. They are included to provide a more complete picture of her profile, as well as to illustrate the complicated nature of brain dementias. Although emotion and cognition have been shown to inextricably link in many ways (e.g. Damasio 1994), this dichotomy is still quite useful and is employed in the psychological and neuroscientific literature. The diagnostic criteria for FTD devised by Neary and colleagues (1998, see Appendix A) are such that four out of five core criteria are descriptive of some kind of self, social, or emotional failure. We shall soon focus on Kelly's social regulatory dysfunctions.

Yet rather than continue to describe these social deficits as neurologists do, an alternative picture is proposed, derived not from inside the clinic but from natural contexts where such interpersonal conduct is made visible. The clinic is a highly structured environment and does not afford many opportunities for dysfunctions in social regulation to reveal themselves. The point here is not to supplant how neurologists learn about and characterize their patients, but to complement their approach with a much more detailed and naturalistic image derived from the traditions of ethnography and conversation analysis.

## A Note on Methods

Conversation analysis (CA) is a unique analytical framework and methodology, somewhat situated between linguistics and sociology, which investigates the micro-organizational practices of interaction (see also Smith, Chapter 3 for further history and explanation). Application of CA to communication and pragmatic disorders is an emerging field and has turned its eyes toward such diverse interactional dynamics as those found with Alzheimer's Disease (Guendouzi and Müller 2006), productive and receptive aphasias (Goodwin 2003), traumatic brain injuries (Body and Parker 2005), split-brain patients (Schegloff 2003) and autism (Wootton 2002).

One reason for the development of this "applied conversation analysis" with patient populations (Schegloff 2003, 28) concerns the ecological validity of the method. As alluded to above, the behavioral picture inside the clinic is a hybrid of synthetic tests, general observations doctors derive from brief interactions, and caregiver reports. CA based on natural video and audio data both grounds and extends this portrayal through meticulously noting the sequential communicative and embodied events from which social interactions are actually composed (but see Avineri, Chapter 5 for application to the clinical setting itself). Using CA outside of the clinic therefore allows one to see subtleties and variations of interactional and pragmatic behavior that controlled experiments do not elicit and clinicians and caregivers are not trained to notice.

The other method this chapter utilizes to study social interaction descends from the tradition of ethnography (Emerson *et al.* 1995; Luhrmann 2000; Fiske 2007). Participant observation (PO) requires that researchers also spend a substantial amount of time in the daily lives of the individuals that they study, not simply observing what they do, but as much as possible participating in those doings as well.

The present chapter demonstrates the value of partnering CA with PO in one major sense—together they provide the analyst with a better radar for extracting characteristic data excerpts. In other words, a truly micro-analytic approach, such as CA, without either quantification over many events or without close familiarity to one's subjects will often cover too narrow a window to pick out case-specific patterns. Through immersion in patients' daily activities and observing them in a variety of contexts one develops a more accurate sense of which behaviors and traits are characteristic or salient. These saliencies can then be contextualized appropriately.

Such an approach becomes especially relevant when construing a subject or their actions as "impaired." There is a certain amount of behavioral variability with everyone, in different social contexts or even at different times of day; it is therefore seeing the temporally extended repetition of certain behaviors that gives the participant observer a sense of if and where the distribution is "skewed," and therefore which data excerpts would illustrate this most accurately. The conclusions drawn from such data analysis, however, sometimes differ from researcher to researcher, and the present chapter is no exception. Taking an unconventional approach, I qualify my particular use of the conversation analytic methodology.

Conversation analysis traditionally rejects overtly psychological descriptions of behavior. Instead, it demands that the analyst direct their attention solely to the visible actualities in an interaction (see Smith, Chapter 3 for theoretical and methodological background). Despite this, Guendouzi and Müller (2006) write that this is not always possible in the context of pathology:

> It can be problematic for someone in clinical research to undertake "pure"
> CA analysis because professional responsibility in diagnosis and interven-

tion relies on a thorough knowledge of patterns of behaviors in pathologies, and therefore, the clinicians will always have prior expectations of what they might encounter in clinical populations. (95) ... clinical researchers adapt CA methodologies to their own purposes... (104).

In the next section I shall adapt the meticulously descriptive eye of CA to posit that Kelly's behaviors demonstrate underlying deficits in the psychological mechanisms necessary for social regulation. I will then examine her brain scans and review some of what we currently know about her particularly atrophied anatomical areas and how they function in a social capacity. Additionally, I suggest that these mechanisms of social regulation are "pre-lingual" and constitute fundamental social proclivities that can manifest as either spoken utterances or embodied actions (Goodwin 2000, 2003). First, however, let us look at how such proclivities actually manifest in a case such as Kelly's.

## Interactions

We turn now to three examples of Kelly behaving in ways that display some dysfunction of social regulation. This claim is further supported by contrasting Kelly's behavior with the actions and reactions of her interlocutors. The examples are chosen to illuminate certain aspects of what is meant by a breakdown in social regulation.

The first discourse data example is spoken, and illustrates something Kelly does frequently, which is turn a conversation topic toward herself. Kelly and Elinor, the director of Kelly's care facility, are visiting the dementia clinic and both they and ethnographers Andrea and Lisa are seated in a hotel room in Westwood. (see Appendix B for transcription notations.)

Immediately preceding line 01, the conversation between Andrea and Kelly

```
    2.1 Chocoholic
    Kelly 13 March, 2007


    01   AND:      my new thing is I'm perfecting
    02             a choc- a: <flourless chocolate cake>
    03                  *---------*--------*-------*((gestural beats))
    04             (0.3)
    05             °that's the thing I've been doing
    06   KLLY:  → well (.) I call myself [a chocoholic
    07   ELIN:                           [flourless
    08   AND:      yea
    09             *--- ((GS's gaze turns toward Elinor))
    10             (0.7)
    11   KLLY:  → I'm a chocoholic
    12             (0.8)((door click off camera, Kelly turns her head))
    13             °sounds like someone's coming
    14   ELIN:     how do you do that. ((Kelly pulls paper from purse))
    15   AND:      u:m what holds it together is actually: egg (.) whites
```

has been about whether or not they enjoy cooking at home. Andrea begins a shift with *my new thing* at line 01 by reporting the dessert she has been *perfecting*. She carefully constructs this utterance to elicit an assessment response from Kelly, and more so to elicit such a response to a single word in her turn. First, Kelly and Andrea were the only participants involved in the prior talk and were then currently seated across from and facing each other, suggesting a mutual, interpersonal orientation (Goodwin, 2000). Second, in line 02 Andrea cuts off the word *chocolate* to insert the adjective *flourless* before it, this adjective being an assessable property of the cake. Third, the restart before the assessable also highlights the importance of the cake being specifically *flourless*. In the American culture of these participants flour is a fundamental ingredient in cake, so one without it is both unique and unusual. Fourth, Andrea further highlights the placement and relevance of *flourless* by accompanying its production with a series of gestural beats (McNeill 1992), which accompany her prosodic accents in line 03. These beats begin with one hand before the repair but add the other at *flourless* to further foreground this word and make salient the phrase in which it is embedded. Fifth, the phrase is temporally stretched for further emphasis.

Following the completion of this carefully constructed turn, an immediate assessment response is expected. Instead, however, there is 0.3 seconds of silence[2] and no change of facial expression from Kelly, indicating a potential lack of uptake. Andrea then quietly attaches an additional utterance in line 05 with the prospective indexical *that*, which, rather than providing new propositional information, condenses what she said to mitigate a possibly face-threatening lack of uptake.

What Kelly does do in line 06, however, is pick up on *chocolate*, the less marked word in Andrea's construction, and *turn the topic toward herself.* Shifting the topic like this is something Kelly does frequently. In fact, after many instances such as this, one gets the impression she is quite egocentric. This is something that has been noted by both her husband and regular caretakers. Among many things that proper social regulation requires is at least a minimal effort to appear equally interested in one's interlocutor as oneself during a conversation (cf. Goffman 1963, 38). During a total of over 20 hours spent with Kelly by the author and other ethnographers she asked them virtually no questions about themselves.

Granted, a declaration such as Kelly's is not unlike Andrea's own comment in lines 01 and 02, informing others about herself and designed in such a way as to expect a reply. For Andrea's utterance to first come off successfully,

---

2.    It is standard practice for conversation analysts to note silences of 0.2 seconds or more as potentially interactionally salient.

however, an assessment uptake should occur immediately afterward. Instead of providing such an uptake, which would show recipiency to Andrea's goal, Kelly begins a new turn by calling herself *a chocoholic*. She even repeats this in line 11 after noting that a lexical repeat by Elinor in line 07 may have audibly covered her own comment.

What Elinor self-selected to say is the type of reaction for which Andrea had designed her turn. Though Kelly and Andrea were in dyadic interaction, the design of Andrea's initial comment so strongly selected for this kind of response that whoever provided it became Andrea's next addressee. In line 09, immediately after the repeat *flourless*, Andrea turns her gaze to Elinor and acknowledges this with *yeah* to follow through with the trajectory she had begun.  As previously noted, it is often what her interlocutors do that serve as contrastable controls for categorizing Kelly's behaviors as "dysfunctional" or "aberrant." By picking up Andrea's course of action, Elinor completed the task that Kelly failed.

Example 2.2 shows a physical action by Kelly that is impulsive, socially disruptive, and shows little evidence of social regulation. On the same day as in example 1, with her husband Bron now present, everyone goes to a local restaurant for dinner. At one point Bron tells Andrea and Lisa a story about an experience he had while in Europe. Kelly can be seen staring at Bron's wine, which is to his left, and then abruptly reaches across him for his glass in the middle of his narrative (see Chapter 7, example 6 for illustration).

Kelly's action displays no consideration of the ongoing social activities in multiple ways:  a) she does not ask for the glass but simply reaches for it; b) she does not look at him before she does so and moves past him as if he was simply an obstacle in her path; c) her timing is insensitive to the structure of the talk Bron constructs, i.e. the initiation of her movement does not occur within any "transition relevance place" in his narrative (Sacks *et al.* 1974); d) her utterance in line 06 is designed not with a politeness formulation (such

```
2.2 Wine Reach
Kelly 13 March, 2007B

01   BRON:     you know I wz just looking for wines
02             and so many wines were over there (in their bottles)
03             but then I [was staying with Italian family and-
04   KLLY:  →              [((reaches across Bron toward his wine; she
05             stops when she bumps into him))
06          → (°give me a taste.)
07   BRON:    OOOooo:hhh ↑wa:it a minu:te.
08   LISA:    he he he he
09   KLLY:    mine's em[pty ((addressed to Andrea))
10   AND:              [you've had two already
11   BRON:    ha ha ha ha
```

as "can you please give..."), but instead as an imperative (*give me...*); e) afterwards, she displays no facial stance of embarrassment of her disruption and provides no apology; and f) the social deviance of this action is made visible by the evaluations all other parties provide; through Bron's extended *OOOooo* in line 07, Lisa's and Bron's laugh tokens in 08 and 11, and the way Andrea's declaration in 10 is phrased with further implication, namely that *[you can't have it because] you've had two already* (Levinson 1983, 97). While any one of these properties may not individually qualify Kelly's behavior as inconsiderate, the assessment of failed impulse control in this social situation derives from their co-occurrence.

In example 2.3 Kelly says and does little relative to those around her, but her *absence* of action speaks volumes. While the analyses of examples 1 and 2 were built around an overt utterance or action, identifying an "error of omission" in the following example appeared at first to be problematic. There are, however, six other participants present who serve as controls, exemplifying behavior one would normally expect in such a situation. When we contrast what they do with what Kelly does we see an unmistakable difference.

The setting this time is in Elinor's office at the care facility. There are a number of others gathered to discuss Kelly's diagnosis and current situation. They are the author (Sam), Bron, Kelly, Rachel (staff), and Elinor. A young assistant, Gina, enters carrying a tray with six glasses of water. As she sets the tray down she bumps it against the table and the glasses tip over and spill.

Everyone, including Kelly, is visibly startled from the crash. Gina is intensely shocked and embarrassed and displays this by covering her face

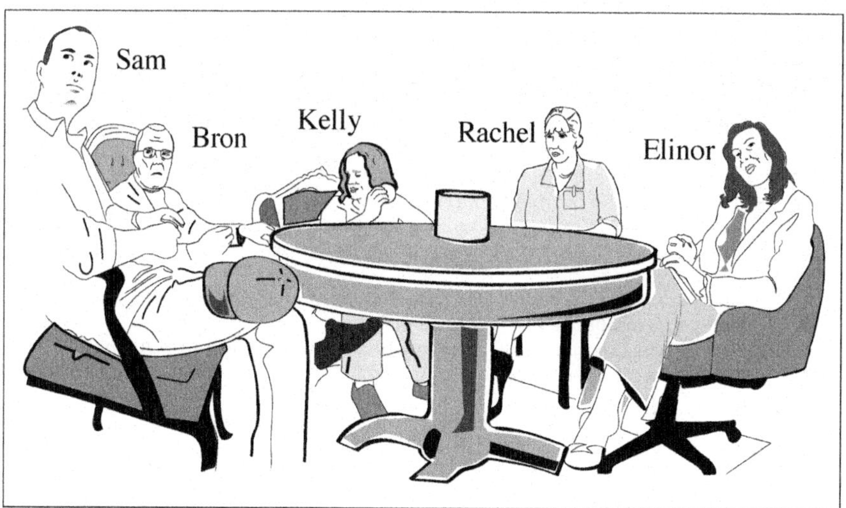


Figure 1.

2.3 Water Spill
Kelly 2/26/07 00:55:15

```
01   ((everyone but Kelly looks at Gina entering room w/ water))
02   ((Gina bumps tray and six glasses crash))
03   BRON:   WHOOOO::::.
04   GINA:   >all right all right all right I'm so:rry<
05           ((covers face))
06    SAM:   it's okay. ((beginning to soak up spilled water))
07           (1.1)
08   GINA:   ooo[:hh
09   ELIN:      [it's jus' water. ((reaches over to pick up
10           glasses))
11           (     ) ((attending to mess))
12   RACH:   he he he he he [heh
13   GINA:                  [oh
14    SAM:   it's [okay. (0.5) I've done that.
15   ELIN:       [it's no problem.
16           (0.5) ((Gina turns around to get something))
17    SAM: → I was a waiter. ((Kelly looking at her cookie))
18   GINA:   sorry. ((whispers as she bumps camera))
19   RACH:   Wake up.
20   GINA:   he he I'm n(h)ot a w(hh)ai [(h)t(h)er.
21   KLLY: →                           [((leans to talk to Bron))
22   BRON:   What?
23           (0.5)
24   GINA:   (that's alright. I'll do [it.)
25   RACH: →                          [that's fine. ((Kelly looks at
26           Bron and her food))
27   GINA:   ohhh
28   ELIN:   this is why it's good you're going into nursing.
29           ((Bron points toward the others to orient Kelly))
30   BRON:   ha h[a ha:
31    SAM:       [>he he he he<
32   GINA:   he he (.) he he
33   ELIN:   that's why I wanted to nurse.
34   GINA:   eh he heh
35   ELIN:   I couldn't do waitressing well.
36   GINA:   I'm fi:ne.
37           (     )
38   ELIN:   (Ok, it's just) water.
39         → ((Kelly stands, watching activity and still eating))
40    SAM:   I've done it with lots of be:er in front of a bunch of
41           gu:[ys
42   BRON:      [(sit down) sit down because it's wet (t's wet)
43         → ((grabs Kelly's purse))
44   KLLY: → how long are we supposed to stay here ((to Bron))
45    SAM:   'n they all like cla:pped, ((gestures clapping hands))
46           'n then I was [like he he he
47                         [((Kelly sits back down))
48   BRON:   yea they will bring the towels and the-
49   GINA:   ugh. (I know I should bring them one by one)
50   BRON:   there we go ((another staff arrives with towel))
51   RACH: → where ya goin. ((looks at Kelly who's stood again))
```

with both hands (for six seconds, through line 13) exclaiming in line 04 >*all right all right all right I'm so:rry*< In the complex series of events that follow, we see two major and perceptively different sequences of activity in parallel: 1) Cooperative efforts among Sam, Bron, Rachel and Elinor to clean the spill and console the embarrassed Gina and 2) Kelly's preoccupation with other activities and goals as Bron attempts to keep her at bay as she tries to leave.

Sam, Rachel, and Elinor immediately set about soaking up the water with napkins and reassure Gina with phrases like *it's okay* and *it's jus' water* (lines 06, 09, 14, 15). Sam tells of a time when he too was embarrassed at a comparable public blunder (lines 14, 17, 40, 45). Elinor jokes with Gina (line 28) at which Sam, Bron, Rachel, and Gina's laughter (lines 30–32) lightens the mood in the room. And finally Elinor shares an experience similar to Sam's in lines 33 and 35. Social psychologists identify such empathetic behaviors as *prosocial*—i.e. those that are "…intended to benefit one or more people other than oneself—behaviors such as helping, comforting, sharing, and cooperation" (Batson 1998, 282).

In contrast, Kelly does not assist with either cleaning the spill or consoling Gina but instead watches the others' activities while eating a cookie (indicated in lines 17, 25, and 39). We know from an earlier sequence that in line 39 Kelly stands up to initiate another attempt to go to her room to check her medicine schedule. Here, however, she is held by Bron, who acts to regulate her actions by physically holding the purse she wears. Kelly's attempts to leave persist through the end of the excerpt, and in line 44 she asks Bron *how long are we supposed to stay here.* Finally, in line 51, Rachel has noticed Kelly getting up again and also attempts to hinder this by asking her where she is going.

Kelly appears oblivious to the social dynamics of the situation and especially its urgency for Gina, essentially displaying no observable concern about what is going on. This does not seem to be a general cognitive obliviousness, however. In other contexts Kelly is able to appropriately respond when addressed and can initiate her own goal-driven behaviors. It therefore appears as if her lack of prosocial action derives from a kind of empathic "blindness" to the major social dimension of this event and a loss of the ability to regulate herself accordingly.

In these examples of Kelly interacting with others we have observed general psychological dysfunctions that might be simplified as egocentricity, a lack of impulse control, and a lack of empathy, all of which have roots in self-regulatory processes that guide proper behavior in social contexts. Before we tap into these processes it will be illuminating to look at the biological basis in Kelly for these dysfunctions.

## Kelly's Brain

We will now identify where in Kelly's brain atrophy has destroyed regions known to support social and socioemotional processing. Figure 2 shows three axial MRI slices of Kelly's brain. The extent of atrophy is quite severe in three major anatomical areas: her temporal poles, orbitofrontal cortex, and medial prefrontal cortex. Scans "A" and "B" are T2-weighted, which makes liquid and pathological tissue appear light and solid material appear dark. We can see in "A" that there are contrasting light areas in the orbits of the eyes and in ventricles filled with cerebral spinal fluid (CSF), which is what is expected from a normal brain scan. The circled regions, however, indicate regions that have essentially disintegrated, most likely from microvacuolation (Snowden *et al.* 1996, 122), and are now replaced with CSF. Slice "C" is a differently weighted scan (without greyscale inversion) that shows structural wasting of the medial prefrontal cortex at this axial level.

Kelly's later scans from 2007 (when ethnographic research was being conducted) were not available for reproduction but were examined by both the author and treating physician who determined that, while greater than before, her pathology had not spread to other anatomical regions and had largely spared her medial temporal lobes (containing hippocampi and amygdalae). While outside the scope of this study, quantification of the precise extent of atrophy would ideally be performed with a technique such as voxel-based morphometry (Bozzali *et al.* 2008) or cortical thickness measurement (Du *et al.* 2007).

## Neuroanatomical Components of Social Regulation

As shown above, the three major brain areas affected in Kelly's brain are her anterior temporal lobes, orbitofrontal cortex, and her medial prefrontal cortex. The field of social neuroscience has strongly implicated these areas in networks supporting social cognition in general and social regulation in particular (see Adolphs 2003 and Beer and Ochsner 2006 for overviews). To explore this further, I begin by reviewing research that has looked specifically at the social functions of these anatomical areas. I will then briefly discuss other connections to Kelly such as the temporal-variant of FTD and issues of sociopathy and development.

### *Anterior Temporal Lobes*

By definition, association cortex—outside primary sensory cortex—synthesizes and manages information from multiple brain areas and serves multiple functions. It has been suggested that the integrative computational demands of such areas make them among the thickest in the brain (Fischl and Dale 2000). It follows that damage to association cortex results in a number of different and even seemingly unrelated cognitive and behavioral deficits.

Some degree of polyfunctionality is certainly the case with Kelly's anterior temporal lobes (also known as the temporal poles or Brodmann's Area 38). The temporal poles (TP), for example, have been strongly connected to both lexical and object meaning as well as face perception. We saw in the behavio-

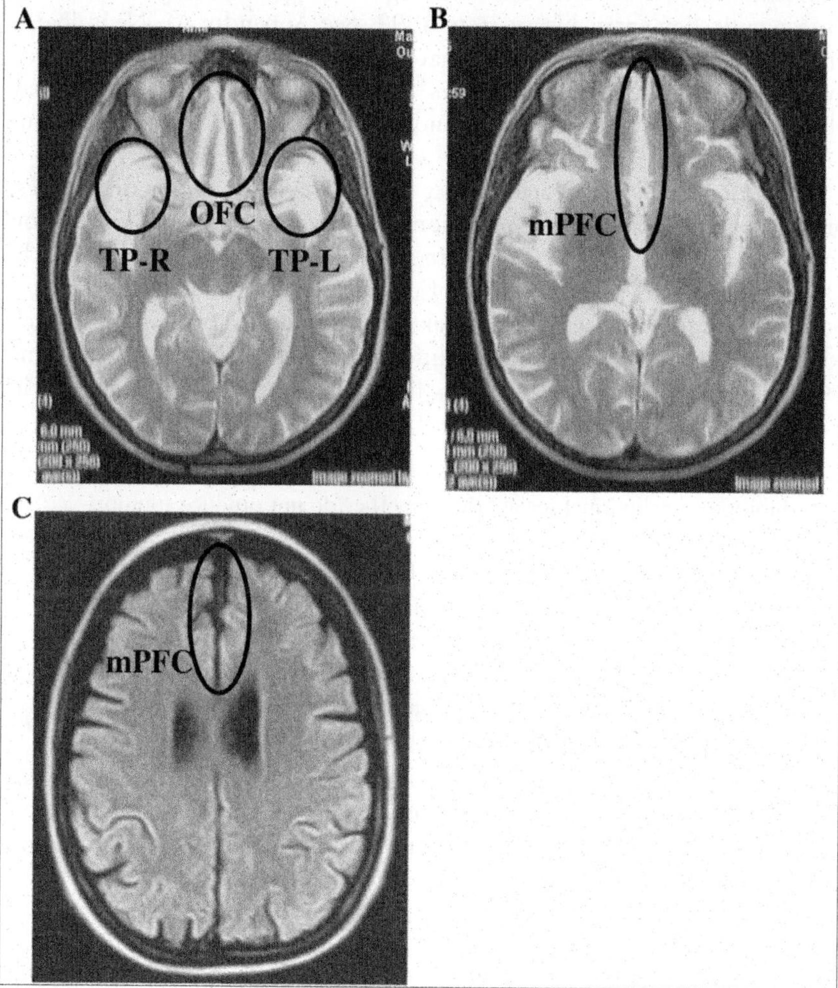



Figure 2.   MRI axial slices of Kelly's brain at increasingly superior planes.  A. T2-weighted scan shows atrophy of orbitofrontal cortex (OFC) and both temporal poles (TP), more pronounced in her right hemisphere (scans in radiological convention).  B. More superiorly, T2-weighted scan shows continued atrophy in TPs as well as along both walls of the medial prefrontal cortex (mPFC). C. More superior still, T1-weighted scan shows continued mPFC atrophy.  Scanned January, 2005.

ral description of Kelly that she has a mix of cognitive and emotional deficits, some of which include these semantic and perceptual abilities. We can begin to account for her co-morbid diagnoses of semantic dementia and prosopagnosia in relation to her damaged temporal poles.

However, even in diagnoses of primary semantic dementia, social behavioral abnormalities are often observed (e.g. the supportive diagnostic criteria for semantic dementia: Neary *et al.* 1998, See Appendix A). Neurologists Snowden, Neary, and Mann write that "Semantic dementia is accompanied by characteristic behavioural changes" (1996, 91) and that "relatives may observe an increasing egocentricity and lack of emotional warmth and concern for others" (1996, 94).

In addition to clinical literature that suggests social processing in the TPs, primatology has also shown this region to be involved in social recognition and behavior (Olson *et al.* 2007). In a review of temporal pole research, Olson *et al.* (2007) note that some of the first indications the anterior temporal lobes were necessary for normal social regulation came from research with non-human primates. The condition known as Klüver-Bucy Syndrome (Klüver and Bucy 1939) results when these regions are bilaterally removed in a monkey.[3] As Olson *et al.* describe:

> Female monkeys with surgical lesions of the TP, excluding the amygdala, exhibit grossly abnormal social behavior. They do not produce appropriate social signals (vocal or facial) nor do they appear to recognize the social signals of peer monkeys. They showed little social interest in their peers, and at times are rejected from their social group... Those with babies are neglectful and often violent towards them, causing consternation among other female monkeys... These findings have been replicated in other species of monkey, suggesting that there is evolutionary conservation of structure-function in the TP across primate species. (Olson *et al.* 2007, 2–3)

Obviously an unethical procedure to perform on humans, the temporal-variant of FTD (tvFTD) might be thought of as nature's cruel equivalent. Olson *et al.* continue their characterization of this region with a comparison of the observed social and emotional deficits in primate TP ablation and human tvFTD (Table 2.1). The similarities are striking.

Further support for the role of the temporal poles in social and emotional processing comes from neuroimaging in humans (Olson *et al.* 2007; Zahn *et al.* 2007). Included in Olson *et al.*'s review was a meta-analysis of nearly 30 different functional MRI and PET studies. Brain imaging meta-analyses provide strong evidence for consistency of activation across multiple and often different experimental paradigms. In a meta-analysis, variability be-

---

3.    Bilateral ablation of the amygdala will also result in this syndrome.

| Monkeys with TP ablation | Humans with right tv-FTD |
| --- | --- |
| Loss of production of facial or vocal signaling | Loss of production of facial expressions; monotone voice |
| Loss of recognition of peer facial or vocal signals | Loss or poor recognition of facial expressions |
| Decreased interest in peers | Self-centered; loss of empathy; preoccupation with non-social stimuli (e.g. jigsaw puzzles) |
| Decreased aggression | Decreased affect |
| Rejection from social group | Avoided by family and friends |
| Decreased status in social hierarchy | Loss of extroversion and social dominance |
| Aberrant and neglectful maternal behavior | -- |
| Aberrant sexual behavior | Hypo or hyper-sexuality |
| Hyperorality | Hyperorality |
| Decreased grooming | Decreased grooming; bizarre changes in dress |

Table 2.1. A list of social and emotional deficits exhibited by monkeys with surgical ablation of bilateral TPs, sparing the amygdala, and the analogous social and emotional deficits observed in humans with right-lateralized tv-FTD. From Olson, *et al.* (2007), with permission.

tween studies gets 'smoothed-over' by the identification of similarly-located clusters of activity. This grouping strengthens claims about regional specificity of functioning. Their meta-analysis found activation peaks in a number of experiments requiring social theory of mind or emotional processing which clustered at the temporal poles.

Anatomically, the temporal poles are massively interconnected with other areas such as the amygdala and hypothalamus (Olson 2007). There is also a large bundle of fibers, the uncinate fasciculus, that reciprocally connects the TPs to another important brain region implicated in social cognition and which is damaged in Kelly: the orbitofrontal cortex.

### Orbitofrontal Cortex

Damage to the orbitofrontal cortex (OFC), on the underside of the prefrontal cortex just above the orbits of the eyes, produced one of the most famous case studies in all of neurological history of a man named Phineas Gage. Formerly polite and dependable, a mining accident in 1849 left Gage with an impolite, crass, and directionless personality. Because his doctor took copious notes and modern scientists have since generated computer simulations of his probable extent of brain damage (Damasio 1994), this case study has had tremendous importance as an initiator of research in brain-behavior relations in social and emotional domains.

We now know that the OFC is quintessential association cortex, and modern research delineates its functionality from a variety of analytical directions and in a number of different ways. One function of the OFC is its contribution to reversal learning, which enables an organism to be flexible to change its appraisals of online stimulus contingencies (Rolls 2006). Presumably this ability is in part necessary for decision-making in social contexts (Schumann 1999). Another function is its contribution to reinforcement learning, which is when an organism learns to associate a particular stimulus with a rewarding or a punishing value. Kringelbach (2005) reviewed research on the OFC and provided a meta-analysis of a large number of fMRI and PET studies to determine where the rewarding or punishing value encoding takes place. He showed a clear geographical distinction (medial vs. lateral) of peak activations during tasks that assessed rewarding or punishing stimuli. Although these descriptive categories may at first appear too broad, social interactions present many occasions in which one can potentially experience "punishing" negative social emotions (such as shame or embarrassment) or "rewarding" positive social emotions (such as pride, amusement, and affiliation). As noted above, some scholars have argued for the fundamental importance of these emotions in motivating social behaviors, such as the work done to maintain face in interaction (Goffman 1967) or sustain social relations over time (Fiske 2002).

Hooker and Knight proposed that the lateral OFC (and extending dorsally to include ventral lateral prefrontal cortex) facilitates "...goal-oriented behavior by inhibiting the influence of emotional information in the context of physical sensation, selective attention, emotion regulation, judgment and decision-making and social relationships" (2006, 307). Following an overview of the OFC's anatomical connectivity, in which they note that it "...has the perfect architecture for modulating neural activity associated with affective information and affectively motivated behavior" (2006, 309), the authors evaluate the possible role of this region in self-regulation in social contexts.

Hooker and Knight cite Beer, whose research has specifically focused on the social-regulatory functions of the orbitofrontal cortex. In an experiment with patients with localized OFC damage, Beer studied the amount and appropriateness of self-disclosure of personal information during an interaction with a stranger (Beer *et al.* 2006). After a structured conversation, she had participants report how they felt the session went. The OFC group significantly differed in how they perceived their social appropriateness relative to how their interactions were later scored by trained judges. While social knowledge of appropriate self-disclosure was preserved among participants, their actual interactions showed otherwise, and they were significantly more prone to inappropriately tease or reveal more personal information to a stranger than were control groups. Incidentally, this notion of an "appropriate" level of self-disclosure based on familiarity with another has a direct counterpart with Kelly. Since the onset of dementia she has developed a few scripted autobiographical narratives that she tells strangers at usually inappropriate moments such as when she had an abortion, or about her brother's suicide.

Moving from the OFC in the medial direction brings one into the anterior, inner surface of the two hemispheres, otherwise known as the medial prefrontal cortex. This is the third anatomical region substantially atrophied in Kelly's brain, and again, research shows this area to be equally relevant to social regulation and social cognition.

### Medial Prefrontal and Anterior Cingulate Cortex

Amodio and Frith (2006) reviewed socially-relevant research on the mPFC and, in another imaging meta-analysis, identified three functionally segregated divisions of the mPFC. Their results strongly suggest that the anterior rostral region (including BA 10) is involved in perception of self and others. On tasks of self-knowledge, person perception, and "mentalizing" (essentially synonymous with theory of mind) peak fMRI and PET activations clustered in this region. Indeed, Iacoboni *et al.* (2004) also found that while watching video clips of actors either alone or in a social interaction, subjects' brain activations increased in dorsomedial prefrontal regions during the latter sequences.

The other mPFC region worth noting in Amodio and Frith's meta-analysis is the posterior rostral region (prMFC), shown to contain almost exclusively activations during "action monitoring" tasks (including BA 8, 9 and 24). They write, "...these findings suggest that conflict monitoring, error monitoring and response selection might depend on a single underlying process instantiated in the prMFC" (2006, 270). This prMFC region may be the area that sounds the alarm, so to speak, when social interactions produce awkward moments, actual or imagined social transgressions, etc. This latter finding also corroborates with well-established cognitive research on an anatomical component of the mPFC—the anterior cingulate cortex (ACC)- that both fMRI and ERP techniques have shown to be crucial to self-monitoring, signaling conflict, and physical pain (Gazzaniga *et al.* 2002, 530). An important extension of this description has recently been made by Lieberman and Eisenberger (2006) who demonstrate that it is not only cognitive conflict and physical pain that activates the ACC, but "painful" social emotions like rejection and ostracism as well.

### Other connections

There is always danger that any case study will lack sufficient relevance for its findings to be generalized. It is for this reason that in the previous three sections I looked toward specific neuroscientific and psychological studies (and meta-analyses thereof) to support speculations about brain-behavior relationships. In addition, clinical evidence from other patients with damage to the same regions as Kelly can also strengthen the hypothesis that the temporal variant of FTD illuminates mechanisms which serve an important role in social regulation. Gorno-Tempini *et al.* (2004) provide a detailed case study of "JT," who exhibited many of the same personality and behavioral changes as Kelly. Like Kelly, JT had a predominantly right-hemisphere-involved temporal variant of FTD. Although the researchers did not analyze JT interacting in social settings, they did perform many neuropsychological tests (such as personality measures) not normally given in the clinic. The results were a compelling quantitative assessment of her behavioral changes. For instance, many of the same qualitative evaluations the present chapter makes regarding Kelly (such as her self-centeredness, lack of empathy, inappropriate self-disclosure, and increasing aggression) also occurred with JT and were substantiated with a variety of controlled measures. Other studies (Rankin *et al.* 2006; Ruby *et al.* 2007) found that this same basic pattern of atrophy correlated significantly with judgments of reduced perspective-taking and empathy made by patients' family members. For example, in Rankin *et al.*, measures were taken across a large number of these patients (N=123) with voxel-based morphometry of MRI-distinguishable brain atrophy. Scores of low empathy and perspective-taking on the Interpersonal Reactivity Index (Davis 1983) correlated most significantly in patients diagnosed with FTD or semantic dementia and contrasted with control groups composed of other neurodegenerative diseases.

Neuropsychiatric patients with frontal and limbic damage similar to Kelly's have fueled other speculations about our social abilities as well. Striking evidence for dysfunction of social regulation, for example, has come from sociopathically aggressive individuals who have engaged in criminal activities (Anderson *et al.* 1999; Mendez 2006; Raine and Yang 2006). While it may seem a stretch to invoke this research in light of the comparatively mild aberrations we witnessed with Kelly, it is important to remember that since her pathology was recognized she has been under watchful eyes in a controlled environment and not allowed to participate in activities which could readily cause harm to others. We do, however, see an increased aggression in recent behaviors, such as kicking or scratching staff and residents at the care facility, and this could be because her atrophy has worsened in the frontal and limbic brain areas implicated in this research.

Making the case for a different resemblance Kelly evokes, however, may prove more compelling. To everyone who knows her, Kelly now seems a little like a child. It is as if her neurodegeneration knocked out those self and social regulatory mechanisms that socialization acts upon in children and she is undergoing a kind of developmental regression. Bron, for example, reported that near the end of her career her interactions with her piano students became more childlike and in an interview one of the staff at Kelly's care facility agreed with this assessment. We also saw in all three excerpts behaviors that could have just as easily been attributed to a young child. It is relevant to note that the prefrontal cortex is the brain region which matures *last* in the ontogeny of the human and does not come fully online with axonal myelenation (speeding information transfer) and the expression of many neurotransmitter receptors until our late teenage years (Diamond 2002; Gogtay *et al.* 2004). Damage to the adult prefrontal cortex may then place the individual "back" in time to when their prefrontal cortex was naturally less developed (see also Joaquin, Chapter 7 for fuller exposition).

## Discussion and Conclusion

Social regulatory processes are a subset of those required for socioemotional competence. We looked at an individual with frontotemporal dementia and observed deficits in both social regulatory processes and socioemotional competence in her everyday interactions. Three of these interactions were detailed using a modified style of conversation analysis, guided in part by participant observation. We then looked into possible causes for her aberrant behaviors by identifying three damaged regions in her brain. Recent research on these anatomical areas was reviewed, and connections were made to the neuropsychological implications of these areas beyond this single case study.

Given the large number of psychological constructs and analogous disorders listed in the previous section, which of these and in what combination would be most helpful to describe Kelly and her behaviors? The question is formidable. Many of the constructs mentioned overlap with each other in as yet unclear ways. This is due simply to the current state of social neuroscience, a vibrant and dynamically changing field. Naturally there are also formidable challenges in determining which cognitive processes are actually present or absent during any observed behavior. In previous sections it was proposed that social regulation is a crucial ability to our social beings and that dysfunction in this domain was likely evident in Kelly's interactions. The associations, however, were self-consciously conjectural, and in actuality go no farther than to simply suggest they are there and that those brain regions were most likely involved, despite an inability to elucidate precise connective mechanisms and causality.

If easy answers are not yet available, we are left instead with an alternative question: why pair CA with the brain in the first place? Neuroscience and neurology speak of behavior, and yet one could say that one does not really know social behavior until one has seen it through a magnifying lens such as CA or a comparable discourse analytic methodology. The interactional richness uncovered is thus far simply unsurpassed by what psychologists, clinicians or caregivers can articulate. With behavior "cut at the joints" in this way then, we can begin a collaboration where the trajectories of both sides squarely face and are much less likely to miss each other. And yet this gap between CA and social neuroscience remains something of an ocean. It will take the collaborative efforts of multiple levels of analysis (some of which may not even exist yet as fields of inquiry) to form an archipelago of steps from one shore to the next. The answer may simply lie in how we explain our research in a language that the next scale of analysis can make sense of and work from. From this an archipelago will slowly but surely form.

## References


Adolphs, R.

2003  Cognitive neuroscience of human social behavior. *Nature Reviews Neuroscience* 4: 165–178.

Amodio, D.M. and C.D. Frith.

2006  Meeting of minds: the medial frontal cortex and social cognition. *Nature Reviews Neuroscience* 7: 268–277.

Anderson, S.W., A. Bechara, H. Damasio, D. Tranel and A.R. Damasio.

1999  Impairment of social and moral behavior related to early damage in human prefrontal cortex. *Nature Neuroscience* 2(11): 1032–1037.

Batson, D.C.

1998  Altruism and prosocial behavior. In *The Handbook of Social Psychology*, edited by D.T.Gilbert, S.T. Fiske and G. Lindzey, 282–316. 4th ed. Oxford: Oxford University Press.

Baumeister, R.F. and T.F. Heatherton

1996  Self-regulation failure: an overview. *Psychological Inquiry* 7(1): 1–15.

Beer, J.S.

2006  Orbitofrontal cortex and social regulation. In *Social Neuroscience: People Thinking about Thinking People*, edited by J. Cacioppo, P. Visser and C. Pickett, 153–165. Cambridge, MA: The MIT Press.

Beer, J.S. and K.N.Ochsner.

2006  Social cognition: A multi level analysis. *Brain Research* 1079: 98–105.

Beer, J.S., O.P. John, D. Scabini and R.T. Knight.

2006  Orbitofrontal cortex and social behavior: Integrating self-monitoring and emotion-cognition interactions. *Journal of Cognitive Neurology* 18(6): 871–879.

Body, R. and M. Parker.

2005  Topic repetitiveness after traumatic brain injury: An emergent, jointly managed behavior. *Clinical Linguistics and Phonetics* 19(5): 379–392.

Bozzali, M., M. Cercignani, C. Caltagirone.

2008  Brain volumetrics to investigate aging and the principal forms of degenerative cognitive decline: a brief review. *Magnetic Resonance Imaging* 26: 1065–1070.

Damasio, A.

1994  *Descartes' error: emotion, reason, and the human brain.* New York: Putnam.

Davis M.H.

1983  Measuring individual differences in empathy: Evidence for a multidimensional approach. *Journal of Personality and Social Psychology* 44(1): 113–126.

Diamond, A.

2002  Normal development of prefrontal cortex from birth to young adulthood: Cognitive functions, anatomy, and biochemistry. In *Principles of Frontal Lobe Function* edited by D. Stuss and R. Knight, 466–503. Oxford: Oxford University Press.

Du, A-T., N. Schuff, J.H. Kramer, H.J. Rosen, M.L. Gorno-Tempini, K. Rankin, B.L. Miller, M.W. Weiner.

2007  Different regional patterns of cortical thinning in Alzheimer's disease and frontotemporal dementia. *Brain* 130: 1159–1166.

Emerson, R.M., R.I. Fretz and L.L. Shaw.

1995  *Writing ethnographic field notes.* Chicago, IL: University of Chicago Press.

Fischl, B., A.M. Dale.

2000  Measuring the thickness of the human cerebral cortex from magnetic resonance images. *PNAS* 97(20): 11050–11055.

Fiske, A.P.

2002  Moral emotions provide the self-control needed to sustain social relationships. *Self and Identity* 1: 169–175.

2007   Learning a culture the way informants do: Observing, imitating, and partici-
       pating. Unpublished manuscript. University of California, Los Angeles.

Gazzaniga, M.S., R.B. Ivry and G.R. Mangun.

2002   *Cognitive neuroscience: the biology of the mind.* 2nd ed. New York: W.W. Nor-
       ton.

Goffman, E.

1963   *Behavior in Public Places.* New York: The Free Press.
1967   *Interaction ritual: Essays on face-to-face behavior.* New York: Doubleday.

Gogtay, N., J.N. Giedd, L. Lusk, K.M. Hayashi, D. Greenstein, A.C. Vaituzis, T.F.
       Nugent 3rd, D.H. Herman, L.S. Clasen, A.W. Toga, J.L. Rapoport, P.M.
       Thompson.

2004   Dynamic mapping of human cortical development during childhood through
       early adulthood. *PNAS* 101(21): 8174–8179.

Goodwin, C.

2000   Action and embodiment within situated human interaction. *Journal of Prag-
       matics* 32: 1489–1522.

Goodwin, C. (ed.).

2003   *Conversation and Brain Damage.* Oxford: Oxford University Press.

Gorno-Tempini, M.L., K.P. Rankin, J.D. Woolley, H.J. Rosen, L. Phengrasamy
       and B.L. Miller.

2004   Cognitive and behavioral profile in a case of right anterior temporal lobe
       neurodegeneration. *Cortex* 40: 631–644.

Gross, J.J.

2001   Emotion regulation in adulthood: Timing is everything. *Current Directions in
       Psychological Science* 10(6): 214–219.

Guendouzi, J. and N. Müller.

2006   *Approaches to Discourse in Dementia.* Mahwah, NJ: Lawrence Erlbaum
       Associates.

Hooker, C.I. and R.T. Knight.

2006   The role of lateral orbitofrontal cortex in the inhibitory control of emotion.
       In *The Orbitofrontal Cortex,* edited by D.H. Zald and S.L. Rauch, 307–324.
       Oxford: Oxford University Press.

Iacoboni, M., M. Lieberman, B. Knowlton, I. Molnar-Szakacs, M. Moritz, J.
       Throop and A.P. Fiske

2004    Watching social interactions produces dorsomedial prefrontal and medial parietal MRI signal increases compared to a resting baseline. *NeuroImage* 21: 1167–1173.

Kaplan, E.F., H. Goodglass and S.Weintraub.

1983    *The Boston naming Test.* 2nd ed. Philadelphia, PA: Lea and Febiger.

Kluver, H. and P. Bucy.

1939    Preliminary analysis of functions of the temporal lobes in monkeys. *Archives of Neurological Psychiatry* 41: 979–1000.

Kringelbach, M.

2005    The human orbitofrontal cortex: linking reward to hedonic experience. *Nature Reviews Neuroscience* 6: 691–702.

Levinson, S.C.

1983    *Pragmatics.* Cambridge: Cambridge University Press.

Lieberman, M.D. and J.H. Pfeifer.

2005    The self and social perception: Three kinds of questions in social cognitive neuroscience. In *The Cognitive Neuroscience of Social Behavior,* edited by A. Easton and N.J. Emery, 195–231. Psychology Press.

Lieberman, M.D. and N.I. Eisenberger.

2006    A pain by any other name (rejection, exclusion, ostracism) still hurts the same: The role of dorsal ACC in social and physical pain. In *Social Neuroscience: People Thinking about Thinking People,* edited by J. Cacioppo, P. Visser and C. Pickett, 167–187. Cambridge, MA: The MIT Press.

Luhrmann, T.M.

2000    *Of Two Minds: An Anthropologist Looks at American Psychiatry.* New York: Vintage Books.

McNeill, D.

1992    *Hand and Mind: What Gestures Reveal about Thought.* Chicago, IL: The University of Chicago Press.

Mendez, M.F.

2006    What frontotemporal dementia reveals about the neurobiological basis of morality. *Medical Hypotheses* 67(2): 411–418.

Neary, D., J. Snowden, L. Gustafson, U. Passant, D. Stuss, B. Black, M. Freedman, A. Kertesz, P.H. Robert, M. Albert, K. Boone, B.L. Miller, J. Cummings, and D.F. Benson.

1998   Frontotemporal lobar degeneration. A consensus on clinical diagnostic criteria. *Neurology* 51: 1546–1554.

Olson, I.R., A. Plotzker and Y. Ezzyat.

2007   The enigmatic temporal pole: A review of findings on social and emotional processing. *Brain* 130(7): 1718–1731.

Premack, D. and G. Woodruff.

1978   Does the chimpanzee have a 'theory of mind'? *Behavioral and Brain Sciences* 4: 515–526.

Raine, A. and Y. Yang.

2006   Neural foundations to moral reasoning and antisocial behavior. *SCAN* 1: 203–213.

Rankin, K.P., M.L. Gorno-Tempini, S.C. Allison, C.M. Stanley, S. Glenn, M.W. Weiner, B.L. Miller.

2006   Structural anatomy of empathy in neurodegenerative disease. *Brain* 129: 2945–2956.

Rolls, E.T.

2006   The neurophysiology and functions of the orbitofrontal cortex. In *The Orbitofrontal Cortex,* edited by D.H. Zald and S.L. Rauch, 95–124. Oxford: Oxford University Press.

Rosso, S.M., G. Roks, M. Stevens, I. de Koning, H.L.J. Tanghe, W. Kamphorst, R. Ravid, M.F. Niermeijer, and J.C. van Swieten.

2001   Complex compulsive behaviour in the temporal variant of frontotemporal dementia. *Journal of Neurology* 248: 965–970.

Ruby, P., C. Schmidt, M. Hogge, A. D'Argembeau, F. Collette and E. Salmon.

2007   Social mind representation: where does it fail in frontotemporal dementia? *Journal of Cognitive Neuroscience* 19(4): 671–683.

Sacks, H., E.A. Schegloff and G. Jefferson.

1974   A Simplest Systematics for the Organization of Turn-Taking for Conversation. *Language* 50(4): 696–735.

Schegloff, E.A.

2003   Conversation analysis and communication disorders. In *Conversation And Brain Damage,* edited by C. Goodwin, 21–55. Oxford: Oxford University Press.

Schumann, J.

1999   A neurobiological basis for decision making in language pragmatics. *Pragmat-*

*ics and Cognition* 7(2): 283–311.

Snowden, J.S., D. Neary and D. Mann.

1996  *Fronto-temporal lobar degeneration: fronto-temporal dementia, progressive apha-sia, semantic dementia.* New York: Churchill Livingstone.

University of California, Los Angeles FTD and Neurobehavior Clinic.

2005–06 Unpublished Outpatient Consultations.

Wootton, A.J.

2002  Interactional contrasts between typically developing children and those with autism, Asperger's syndrome, and pragmatic impairment. *Issues in Applied Linguistics* 13(2): 133–159.

Zahn, R., J. Moll, F. Krueger, E.D. Huey, G. Garrido, and J.F. Grafman.

2007  Social concepts are represented in the superior anterior temporal cortex. *PNAS* 104(15): 6430–6435.

# — 3 —

# Exploring the Moral Bases of Frontotemporal Dementia through Social Action

Michael Sean Smith

## Introduction

Since its earliest descriptions, frontotemporal dementia has been captured most saliently by the social and moral degradation it causes in the afflicted persons. From today's perspective, it is striking how prejudiced some of these descriptions are, as in Jung and Solomon (1993) who reference an early investigator, Sadler who in 1945, "...quaintly noted that patients with [FTD] 'are morally loose, and lie, steal, squander their money, and drink'" (195). The distance we see today from remarks like "morally loose" in neurological and psychiatric description—evident even in Jung and Solomon's use of "quaint" for Sadler's remarks—is the result of the fields' maturation where instead of simply naturalizing these assessments, the attempt now is to explain what it is they are assessing. As a result, today we see slightly more distanced descriptions like "early decline in interpersonal and personal conduct," "disinhibited speech and gestures,' and 'loss of emotional warmth, sympathy, and indifference to others" (Neary *et al.* 1998; cf. appendix A).

As it should be clear, even these criteria are rooted somewhere phenomenologically closer to others' perceptions of FTD, than to the pathology "as it is," which understandably remains difficult to isolate. Because the pathology's socio-behavioral disturbances manifest over time and are often coupled with the patient's lack of insight, they are often most clear to those who share a history with the patient, often necessitating a greater role for caregivers or informants in diagnosis in helping complete behavioral inventories (c.f., Introduction, this volume). The dependency on others' descriptions in diagnosis have not limited our neuropsychiatric understanding of FTD. Some studies using adjective scales (e.g., "coldhearted," "dis-social," "calculating," etc.) given to caregivers for describing the patient, have found them useful in disassociating FTD from other dementias, discriminating behavioral phenotypes, as well as demonstrating the co-morbidity of its different symptomatic expressions (Rankin, Baldwin, Pace-Savitsky, Kramer, and Miller, 2005; Rankin, Kramer, and Miller, 2005; Rankin *et al.* 2003; Rankin *et al.* 2004). Others' perceptions then seem to have some systematic relation to FTD's behavioral, if not neurobiological, disorder.

Though neither the behavioral inventories or the adjective scales are often characterized as moral assessments, questions that ask caregivers whether the patient 'shows socially embarrassing behavior' (Cambridge Behavioural Inventory, problem 49; Bozeat *et al.* 2000) or is "extremely unsympathetic" or "cold hearted" (Interpersonal Adjective Scale, rating 8 on adjectives 90 and 92 respectively; Mychack *et al.* 2001) presuppose that the attributes are morally dispreferred. Negative assessments, like "embarrassing," "indifferent," "coldhearted," "calculating," etc., function in everyday use as social sanctions, which Erving Goffman points out, are essentially "norms about norms," or prescriptive actions given to society members to punish another's behavior for its failure to adhere to a prescriptive norm that they all presumably hold in common. Neither the sanction nor the norm, Goffman continues, are significant for their "...intrinsic, substantive worth but in what they proclaim [but not necessarily determine] about the moral status of the actor" insofar as he or she is expected and is able to conform (1971, 95). These moral assessments are generally poor indicators of the individual or his or her behaviors, irrespective of other considerations, but rather seem to index more the perceiver, and how the particular behavior affects him or her. As such, the "morality" of these assessments should therefore not be taken to be an attribute of the pathology, but of its saliency in others' phenomenological apperception. Simply capturing others' perceptions of the dementia is, however, still a step removed from what could be described as its aesthetically "pure" description of FTD in-of-itself, a fact of which no doubt motivates current attempts to find models, cognitive or affective, that rely as little as possible on informant description in explaining FTD's pathology.

In spite of the qualifications given above, or current attempts at lessening their need, the morality of these descriptions remains something endemic to FTD as it appears in the patient and others' social world and thus may be of theoretical and possibly therapeutic benefit to explore. For instance, recent studies have begun suggesting that FTD results in a "moral agnosia" (Mendez, Anderson and Shapira 2005), a loss in moral reasoning, or in a "acquired sociopathy" (Mendez 2006; Mendez, Chen, Shapira and Miller 2005; Rankin *et al.* 2008). However, there has yet been a critical analysis as to how and when the patients' behavior is merely problematic and where instead it is morally transgressive, or how others' moral assessment of the patient develop from or contribute to this in everyday interaction. The purpose of this chapter is to determine if FTD does cause a breakdown in the moral order of interaction, and if so, examine how that occurs procedurally through others' actions in relation to the patients. Before attempting this, it will be necessary to discuss the assumptions for how morality will be expected to appear in the data and the limits and strengths of the analysis.

## Background

### *Garfinkel and the breaching tasks*

A unique perspective on morality comes from Harold Garfinkel's early sociological experiments, or what are better known as his "breaching tasks" (Garfinkel 1963; Heritage 1984a, 78–102). The earliest was the tic-tac-toe task, where experimenters (E) were instructed to initiate a game of tic-tac-toe with a subject (S) offering them the first move. Afterwards, E was instructed to erase the S's mark, place it elsewhere, and then place his or her own mark, all without hinting that anything extraordinary had occurred. The Ss' reactions split them into two distinct groups: most Ss protested and demanded an explanation from E, while the rest showed little disturbance, acted as if E was joking, or, interestingly, thought a "new game" was occurring (Garfinkel 1963, 206; summarized from Heritage 1984a, 78–79). When Garfinkel looked at the intensity of the Ss' reaction, he found that those who showed the most frustration did so because they tried to "normalize the [E's] discrepancy" while still using tic-tac-toe as the constituent order; E's moves were only sensible then as violations. Those Ss who showed the least disturbance, however, took the Es' move as the new constituent order and abandoned tic-tac-toe as the meaningful precondition. When Garfinkel manipulated breaches in more socially natural contexts, he found that the same operations also applied in these contexts and that it was more the lack of meaningful interpretation that led to hostility and not necessarily the breach itself. The reactions seen in natural contexts were much stronger and more toxic. Ss immediately became "righteously hostile" (Heritage 1984a, 81), demanded explanations, and strongly sanctioned the Es' behavior as "mean, inconsiderate, selfish, nasty, and impolite" (Garfinkel 1963, 226). The breaches occurring in these contexts left little room for the subjects to treat them as anything other than threatening.

The regularity of the reactions suggested to Garfinkel that the relationship between the "normative regulation of action" is not dependent on the sanctity of the social norm, if that could even be identified, but on actors' expectations for "the stability of concerted action." (Garfinkel 1963, 198, in Heritage 1984a, 83). This suggests that the relationship between transgression, moral order, and sanctioning is a procedural one in which an actor only becomes morally sanctioned if and when his or her actions resist normalization while preserving the prior stability of the interaction. Normative regulation, i.e., sanctioning or punishing the actor, then is not distinct from non-normative regulation but simply the severest means by which interactants maintain normalcy. Though unusual, it is not completely unexpected that the subjects, once reaching this point, frequently treated the experimenters' breaches as purposeful and specifically directed at the subjects, or in some cases, without knowing their true purpose, even constructed motivations for the experimenters "out of whole cloth" (Heritage 1984a, 99). Being "righteously hostile" towards the actions of another is certainly facilitated in "knowing" he or she is acting with malicious intent or from a morally inferior position. The fact that the interpretations of the experimenter were occasioned by the breach and to varying degrees fabricated by the subject makes their expression all the more remarkable as it suggests that while moral conflict may be dyadic, triadic, quadratic, etc., its moral assessment may be entirely monadic. The usefulness of Garfinkel's 'procedural morality' is in first demonstrating that transgressions are not given in any situation but necessarily develop through it, and from this makes it possible to analyze how disruption or transgression occurs, not by presupposing its violation, but by how it is constructed by the patients' co-participants.

### *Conversation analysis—a non-cognitive approach*

In investigating normative functioning in FTD, it is necessary to determine what can and cannot be the target of the analysis. Conversation analysis (CA) takes as its task to "render the empirical analysis answerable to the specific details of the research materials" (i.e., audio/video recordings of participants talking in interaction) (Heritage 1984a, 234). This excludes any a priori prescriptive or proscriptive limit on the relevancy of any point in the data and only selects constructs that are empirically identifiable and relevant for the data at hand. As Levinson (2000, 295–296) points out, this results "in a strict and parsimonious structuralism and a theoretical asceticism…[where]…the emphasis is on the data and patterns recurrently displayed therein.' Since the data is from recorded interactions, the analyses focuses on the public motivation and effect of actions and not the private, psychological constructs are generally excluded except when evident in the data. This leads some researchers to describe CA as an inherently non-cognitive approach (Potter 2005: 743). If CA is analytically agnostic about the mental states of normal participants, however, the question that remains is what are we learning about FTD, as a neuropathology, when using CA?

One reason CA focuses on the public nature of action stems from its particular mode of analyses. Analyses of actions or turns-at-talk are done against the "next-turn proof procedure" where the successive production of each turn incrementally confirms the participants' (and analyst's) interpretation of a prior turn (Hutchby and Wooffitt 1998, 15; c.f. also Sacks *et al.* 1974). One limitation in the FTD data, however, is the patients and their co-participants rarely seek a consensus on the meaning of a prior action. This leads analysts in this volume to employ modified approaches. One approach is to compare an action found in a sequence in the FTD data against similar type of action found in general interaction (ex. 01 from the current chapter is an example of this). Another approach is to compare co-participants' actions that are concurrent with, as opposed to next after, the patients, especially when both actions are directed to the same object (excellent examples of this can be seen in Torrisi, Ch. 2, and Mikesell, Ch. 4, in this volume). As a result, this research relies primarily on the co-participants' analyses of the patient, and not the patients' internal view. Rather than being an artifact of the analysis, this can be seen as the result of both the co-participants' expectations and the patients' situated participation in the interactions.

## Participants

The participants of this study are Louise and Vera, aged 79 and 72, who were diagnosed with the behavioral variant of FTD. Louise lived with her two adults daughters, Jess and Dana, and was diagnosed almost ten years prior with distributed atrophy in her right dorsolateral prefrontal cortex (Smith, 29 August, 2003: fieldnotes). She presented with difficulties in initiative, attention, short-term memory, and some behavioral problems. Vera lived at home with her husband, had adult children living nearby, grandchildren, and a full time caretaker, Bonnie. Both of her anterior temporal lobes were significantly affected, with greater involvement in the left than right. In addition, it was also suggested that structures medial to the temporal lobes such as the orbitofrontal cortex were also atrophied (Mendez, Chen, Shapira, Lu, Miller 2006, 103; Smith, 11 November, 2003: fieldnotes). She was described as disinhibited, lacked empathy, and had a developed anomia or semantic dementia (c.f. Introduction, Chapter 1, this volume). The patients were very different in their presentations and conduct. Louise was mostly personable if sometimes detached from interaction and any difficulty she did cause was often subtle and transitory. Vera, however, was more autonomous, assertive, and less likely to follow others' lead. As a result, she required more scrutiny and frequently drew (and sought) the attention of others in public. In addition, as will be important later, while Louise showed more interest in the ethnography's aims, Vera seemed less interested in either the study or my presence (as will be shown though, this initial assessment is less than accurate). Despite their differences, their participation comes to influence the interactions in remarkably similar ways.[1]

## Analysis

The data in this study suggest that a systematic alteration occurs in the interactions with FTD patients as seen through the patient's co-participants' use of recurrent practices which both identify problems in the patients' participation and attempt to alter the patients' participation. One set of practices is attempts at prompting the patients' involvement in the interaction. These practices become especially noticeable because they are used with both patients and are deployed similarly across the data. In excerpt 3.1, we see four turns produced by Bonnie towards Vera during a meal at which I was also present.[2]

In CA, Bonnie's turns are called assessments that are produced in first position (not as responses) to Vera, the recipient. Prior work on assessments suggests that they overwhelmingly engender second assessments from recipients and serve important interpersonal functions (C. Goodwin 2003; Goodwin and Goodwin 1992; M.H. Goodwin 1980; Heritage 2002; Heritage and Raymond 2005; Pomerantz 1984; Raymond and Heritage 2006). Bonnie also tags Vera's name to three out of the four turns (lines 01, 04, and 09), thereby selecting Vera and not Michael as the next-speaker. While Vera does nod (though gives no response after line 07), she never looks up during the assessments nor displays an appreciation for the assessments, thus effectively shutting down the appreciative engagement that Bonnie is pursuing.

The absence of Vera's seconds, however, is less significant than the repetition of Bonnie's firsts. Bonnie, looking at Vera during the assessments, sees that Vera's responses are perfunctory, indicating that a subsequent elaborated response from Vera would be unlikely. Bonnie never substantially redesigns the assessments, nor immediately re-pursues seconds from Vera or Michael,

---

1.  "Participation" (Goffman 1981) is a significantly different way to speak of the individual than is using "behavior." Participation includes a description of the target behavior (simple or complex movement, utterance(s), and/or absence thereof), *and* a description of how others' behavior relates to it. As such, any description, value, or classification of the target behavior will always take others' prior and/or next behaviors into account.

2.  In many of the examples below, I am a participant in the interaction. In the analysis, however, I will often refer to myself in third-person.

```
3.1 Bonnie's Assessments
Vera, 11 December, 2003D

01   BONN    The::se are good Ve^ra,
02   VERA    ((nods head up and down))

03           ((Time & text omitted))

04   BONN    Is your soup goo^d Vera,
05   VERA    ((nods head up and down))

06           ((Time & text omitted))

07   BONN    These are so::: good,

08           ((Time & text omitted))

09   BONN    This is so:: good Ve^ra,
10   VERA    ((nods head up and down))
```

suggesting that the second assessment may have not been the primary goal. Bonnie does, however, produce her assessments after gazing at Vera who is noticeably disengaged from the interaction. This timing suggests that the assessments are more contingent on the lack of sustained talk with Vera, and therefore, not seeking a specific response or perhaps any response, but simply seeking to reengage Vera into the interaction. Overall, Bonnie's actions displayed her concern for the current disengagement and selected Vera as its source. The way in which Bonnie constructs her assessments in particularly telling in this regard: exempting Michael while selecting Vera in the turn-construction effectively identifies both who is and who is not accountable for this disengagement. A similar attempt to encourage Vera's participation can be seen in the next excerpt, 3.2. Vera, her daughter, Susan, and I are seated at a restaurant table. Susan notices that I ordered the same soup as Vera and announces it to Vera.

Susan's *Oh look, Mom...* in line 01 focuses Vera's attention through its semantics, high volume, and pitch. Speakers often produce *Oh* when hearing something unanticipated, and upon hearing it, display their 'change of state' to others (Heritage 1984b). Here, Susan uses it to alert Vera to what she will subsequently direct her towards. Her next turn constructional unit (TCU), *Michael just ordered what you're having,* announces the prior event explicitly referencing Vera and Michael. Vera's uptake in line 03, *Oh,* is quick and mirrors Linda's prior in volume and pitch. She then stops and initiates an insert sequence asking Susan *what is this, honey?* (likely a complication of her anomia) (Schegloff 2007, 99). After the insert sequence, Vera then produces an assessment to Michael, *Oh, isn't just a wonder of the world, honey* in lines 06 and 07.

```
3.2 Clam Chowder
Vera, 11 November, 2003

((Family is sitting in restaurant and Michael has just ordered clam
chowder, which is the same item that Vera ordered))
01   SUE     ^Oh look^ Mom, Michael just^ ordered what you^'re
02           having
03   VERA    ^Oh ((Turns to Susan)) ^What is this honey^?
04              ((Pointing to bowl))
05   SUE     Clam chowder
06   VERA    ((Nods; Turns to Michael)) Oh isn't just a wo::nder of
07           the wor:ld honey?
08   MICH    Mm mh
```

In the end, Susan's prompt facilitates Vera's participation towards another
co-participant, and in doing so Vera is able to maintain that trajectory through
five turns of talk, the insert sequence, the different roles selected (speaker—
recipient), and produce more than just agreement but a fully elaborated action to that co-participant. Susan's actions are more elaborate (and successful)
than Bonnie's in ex. 01, but the issue they addressed are the same, namely the
patients' disengagement. A similar event occurs with Louise as well in excerpt
3.3. This excerpt begins when I ask Jess a question. Jess initiates a response,
seems to expand on it, but then stops in line 05.

Jess's response to Michael in lines 03 to 05 is constructed as ongoing turn,
as shown by her rise in pitch at the end of the TCU in line 04 and the list-
like format of her TCUs (Jefferson 1991; Selting 2007). At the beginning
of line 05, however, Jess looks to Louise who had been looking at Dana and
Michael. Here, Jess noticeably raises her pitch and volume through line 05
while holding her gaze on Louise. Coming just prior to Jess's summons in line
07, this suggests that Jess is working to get Louise's attention at a point in
the talk she expects to have relevance for Louise. When Jess prompts Louise,
she first summons her with *Mom* in line 07 and then makes the announce-

```
3.3 Monty
Louise, 10 September, 2003B

01   MICH    Did you guys own a dog when you were in
02           Georgia? ((To JESS))
03   JESS    Mm mh ((Louise's eye gaze disengages))
04   JESS    His name was Montague, he was an
05           Australian shepard^, ((eye gaze shifts to
06           Louise))
07   JESS    Mom^ (0.8) Michael asked about Monty^
08   LOIS    Oh:::^ my:::
09   JESS    Wasn't he a good fella?
10   LOIS    Yeah::: he was a good ol' dog ((finishes with
11           eye gaze directed to Michael))
```

ment *Michael asked about Monty*. The summons in of itself carries a specific presupposition about the recipient, or as Charles Goodwin argues, "the use of a summons to someone who is only a couple of feet away...is clearly dealing not with issues of mere [physical] co-presence...but rather of alignment to the activity being pursued by the summoner" (2007, 64) Louise's first response in line 08, *oh my*, treats the announcement as newly received, suggesting that she was indeed disengaged from that prior activity. After Jess's assessment in line 09, Louise's next response *Yeah, he was a good ol' dog* contains both an agreement to Jess and a response to Michael to whom she turns towards at the end of the turn.

Jess's interrogative assessment in line 09 is informative because it reveals Jess's reasoning for her abandoning the prior turn in line 5 and her prompt for Louise. Prior to line 09, Jess reformulated the generic reference, *dog*, into *Montague* and at that point looks towards Louise, and in doing so marks the moment when Louise's lack of participation becomes relevant. Jess's announcement then presents *Monty* as an unmarked assessable whose simple production is expected to secure Louise's alignment (Goodwin 2007). Once establishing Louise's recognition, Jess takes this opportunity to reminisce with Louise with *wasn't he a good fella?* Comparing the referent for the prompt in this excerpt to the referent, *clam chowder*, in ex. 02 which was not treated as having any elaborated meaning, we can see how here, in ex. 03, *Monty* is significant not only for making an immediate connection but a personally historical one as well.

Altogether, these excerpts show the caregivers deploying specific practices in the attempt to alter what was problematic about the interactions, namely the conflict between the co-participants' expectation of an active engagement and the patients' current disengagement. Bonnie's actions from excerpt 01 suggest that this is a common concern whenever the patient is present but not actively speaking. Similarly, Susan's actions in excerpt 02, though more ambitious, are also directed at getting the patient to orient to her interpersonal environment. Jess's actions in excerpt 03, however, demonstrate how acutely, here being related to a specific referent, *Monty*, this disengagement can be perceived

Erving Goffman (1972, 64, in Goodwin 1986, 286) noted that the most ubiquitous feature in interaction is the way in which "two or more persons in a social situation ... jointly ratify one another as authorized co-sustainers of a single, albeit moving, focus of visual and cognitive attention." Talk and interaction, and indeed sociality, require both the participants' practical means and interest in establishing and reproducing that joint attention. In these interactions, the co-sustained focus of attention is seldom assumed by the caregivers and is often more the product of their deliberative actions. This is important; generally in face-to-face interaction, unless one is the recipient of a prior, the decision *not to talk* is treated as much a prerogative as is the decision *to talk*. The unexceptional production of the prompts then, as well as the patients' not treating them as invasive, seems to speak to an overall change that has occurred in the patients' participation relative to others' expectations. Most importantly though, these prompts are neither directed to random events, nor every event, but only to those that connect the patient with others: shared activities, shared likes, and shared memories. These practices though, are not always successful in altering the patients' participation towards another; in the last excerpt analyzed in this paper involving Vera, we will see a prompt that has limited effect.

There are many situations in which the patients' disruptive participation, rather than their lack of participation, is treated as problematic. FTD patients often act in a way that others find objectionable or inappropriate and often show a disregard for others' wants or feelings (Miller *et al.* 1997). When the patients' actions become disruptive to others' courses of action, the co-participants would instead use practices that actively suppress or modify the patients' participation relative to their own. A subtle expression of this can be seen below in excerpt 3.4 where Louise, her daughters, and I are traveling by car, when Jess starts telling me of their recent medical visits.

When Louise begins talking in line 03, Jess was producing a list showing her turn to be ongoing (Jefferson 1991; Selting 2007). Prior to that, the interaction was in what Schegloff and Sacks (1973) call an incipient state where a lull in the talk was in effect just prior to Jess's turn. This along with

```
3.4 Goatee
Louise, 07 October, 2003A

01   JESS    So we've been down at UCLA a lot with the dentist, and
02           the cardiolo[gist, and the-
03   LOIS                [Are you trying to grow a beard?
04   MICH    Huh?
05   LOIS    Are you trying to grow a beard?
06   MICH    Uh::: Just a little goatee
07   LOIS    Huh?
08   MICH    Justa little goatee
09           (0.8)
10   MICH    So you went to go see the dentist? ((To JESS))
11   MICH    ((Starts to rub chin))
12   LOIS    Itches ((To Michael))
13   MICH    Heh heh heh
14   DANA    The dentist, (the) regular doctor, the [cardiologist=
15           (xxxx) (xxxxxx)
16   LOIS    ((To Michael))                          [Na:::h, you're
17           too good lookin to hide your face with a beard
18   MICH    heh heh heh he(h)
```

Jess's *so* prefacing suggests that she was proffering a topic for Michael's possible expansion and thus projecting an extended course of action (Bolden 2006; Schegloff 2007, 169). Louise's question to Michael in line 03 thus subverts 1) her daughter's immediately on-going turn, 2) its course of action, and 3) Michael's role as Jess's recipient. After his response to Louise, Michael attempts in line 10 to renew Jess's topic by recycling her prior *so* and *the dentist*. Nevertheless, Louise restarts in line 12 and does so again after lines 16 and 17, where Dana also attempts to renew Jess's telling by recycling *the dentist*. Michael and Dana's recycling supports Jess's course of action through format-tying or by tying back, over Louise's turns, to others' prior turns (Sacks 1967 in M.H. Goodwin 1990, 177). This practice publicly selects whose actions are ratified and effectively suppresses Louise's participation vis-a-vis others.

The extent that Louise's actions relate to "disinhibition," can best be described through her gaze shifts. During Jess's turn, Louise looks towards Michael, looks away, and then abruptly looks back (doing what would be called a "double-take"), shortly before her question. In general interaction, when speakers want to say something new, there is often only a small window for that to occur. For the co-participants here, that window began closing as the trajectory of Jess's talk became evident. Louise's utterances, however, always seemed to be synchronized with her initial noticing, and thus without consideration of these interpersonal or temporal constraints; this was true even when her co-participants enforced these expectations.

This format tying in essence deconstructs the patient's participation relegating it to background or interference. It is important to note that this is not an arbitrary decision on the co-participants' part but is co-ordinated on the in/congruity of the patients' actions. A simpler way to characterize the practice is to say the co-participants are trying to "ignore" the disruptions either by the simply talking over the patient or waiting until the patients finishes before continuing. This is something that co-participants also do with the patients' non-verbal offenses, like spitting out food while eating in a diner or grabbing food off others' plates (Smith, 11 November, 2003: field notes). The co-participants maintained order by not commenting on the behaviors: that is, a "non-response" seemed to be an attempt to prevent the patients' behavior from disrupting what was their current activity.

There are many situations, however, that the patients' action so radically transform the prior context, however, that ignoring it is neither possible or desirable. In excerpt 3.5, Vera, Bonnie, Vera's friend Diane, and I walk into a local antique store, where a few feet ahead of us, stand a young couple browsing the merchandise. As Vera walks by the man from behind, she reaches up around his back and taps his shoulder opposite her side, playing a practical joke that children often do with the intention of causing the target to look towards the side opposite the joker. The man does not move, but the woman walks away from Vera while laughing and grabbing the man's arm.

There are numerous ways that Vera transgress expected norms of conduct: touching a stranger, showing unwarranted familiarity, calling him munchkin and honey (likely also due to her anomia as I was similarly referred to as "munchkin" or "little boy"). Diane immediately treats this as problematic saying to Bonnie in line 10 *you handle this* before walking away. Vera's next turn, *You want to know something? The people down here got this one, and it is a wonder of the world* is recognizable as a positive assessment, but what it assesses and why are difficult to interpret at face value. After Vera walks away, Bonnie steps toward the couple and says in lines 15 to 17, *Yeah, this is the same store as the [store name] down there. Have you been in that store?* More than just reformulating Vera's ambiguous references (F: *this one* > W: *this is the same store*; F: *the people down here* > W: *as the [store name] down there*), Bonnie also prefaces it as an agreement to Vera's prior assessment and ends it by asking the woman *have you been in that store?* The woman aligns with this course of action in her *no* response and provides an account we've just noticed this one. Bonnie responds with a *wow*-prefaced turn that treats the woman's response as notable and in need of resolution for which Bonnie provides with directions to the other store.

This outcome does not imply that Bonnie truly made Vera's breach disappear. In lines 23 to 26, Diane confesses to Michael that Vera's trespasses

```
3.5 Munchkin
Vera, 11 December, 2003A


07   VERA    [you're a little munchkin honey ((to man))
08   BONN    [heh heh heh
09   DIAN    [heh heh heh
10           you handle this ((to Bonnie))= ((Diane walks away))
11   VERA    =you want to know something. the people down [here,=
12   XXX                                                  [(xxxxx)
13   VERA    =got this one and it is a wonder of the world
14           ((Vera moves away from the couple))
15   BONN    yeah this is the same store as the (name) (down).
16           there
17           have you been in that store,
18   WOMN    nuh huh: we just (of) noticed this one,
19           we haven't even noticed (that before)
20   BONN    wo::w,
21           go down the way, and on that side of street
22           [(     ) (continued; camera moves away)
23   DIAN    [that's what she does an- and it doesn't bother her,
24           that's why she's so great.
25           it just drives me crazy.
26           i'm going ^o:h ^my: g^o:d
```

[drove her] *crazy*. Nor did this necessarily occur for the couple, who more likely just accepted what was convenient. Their concerted actions, however, show that normality is the preferable order they tacitly agree to even if marginalizing what had just occurred. Like Garfinkel's research, this excerpt shows that enforcing the actor's compliance with the prior order is only one way to normalize the situation. Here, Bonnie provides an alternative script for how the couple should reinterpret Vera's actions and, in doing so, re-constitutes a new framework that is markedly different from the one left after Vera's prior turn.

## Co-participant Practices and Moral Assessments

Similar to the subjects in Garfinkel's breaching studies, the patients' co-participants constantly evaluate the interactions in relation to their presuppositions for the stability or normalcy of the talk. Overall, the practices seemed to follow three trajectories: either after noting the patients' disengagement, the co-participants 1) select the patient as next speaker and reformulate the just prior talk or activity so as to invite the patient's observance of the prior framework (ex. 01–03), or if the patient breaches an interaction, the co-participants then 2) select a prior or other co-participant as next speaker and reformulate the talk so as to support the talk prior to the patient's breach (ex. 04), or if the patient breaches an interaction with an individual who was not part of the prior interaction, the co-participants 3) reformulate the patients' prior actions and selects the other individual as next speaker for re-constituted order. The first two practices work to maintain a prior order either by encouraging the patient to conform to expectations or by attempting to prevent the patient's participation to the current activity. The third strategy, exemplified by Bonnie's actions in excerpt 05, *Munchkin*, best represent the practice Garfinkel found to produce the least frustration: abandoning the prior order, normalizing the potential breach, and re-constituting a new order. There, Bonnie simply interprets Vera's prior turn, treats it as unproblematic, and produces the reformulated action towards the couple without hesitation. In contrast, Diane's response in lines 23 to 26 shows frustration at Vera's breach precisely because of Diane's insistence on using her interpretation of the prior condition (i.e., not talking to or touching strangers; not referring to them with diminutive references; not producing incoherent talk, etc.) as the sole means for interpreting the Vera's action.

The reader can notice that the moral hostility documented by Garfinkel is largely absent from these excerpts. This does not mean that it does not occur, but when it does, it was often in dyadic situations, similar to the two following excerpts (3.6, 3.7). In the first, involving Dana and Louise, the family is discussing the events surrounding the death of Louise's husband, when

```
      3.6 'You can't erase everything'
      Louise, 10 September, 2003A

      01  LOIS   But Dad died when I was up here (in California)
      02  DANA   Dad died- you were living with him in
      03         Georgia
      04         We brought him to the hospital in Boston
      05  DANA   [Remember, you stayed at the apartment=
      06  LOIS   [Tha::t's right tha:::t's right
      07  DANA   =on tw- twenty-fourth street [while=
      08  LOIS                               [Yeah yeah yeah
      09         You're right
      10  DANA   =he was- at- at- at- Boston medical center
      11  LOIS   That's where he died right
      12  DANA   There you go
      13  LOIS   You know it's- it's- I erased it
      14         (0.8)
      15  LOIS   I don't like to remember
      16
      17  DANA   Yeah but you rememb- but you- but I mean
      18         you can't erase everything Mom
      19  LOIS   No::::: but the details- Like you know,
      20         I got married, I had babies,
      21         I had your father, Your father died.
      22
      23         (that's-) you know [(xxxx)-
      24  DANA                      [There was a lot of
             time in between that Mom
```

Louise 'misremembers' the place of his death.

The import here is not merely that Dana displays her offense at Louise's *faux pas*, but that she does so by pressing her point beyond Louise's earliest concession (line 06), and whereas Louise initially only provides only one such gaffe, Dana now expands that into multiple ones (lines 02–04, 05, 07, and 10), to which Louise gives numerous confirmations (lines 06, 08–09, and 11) before being acknowledged with Dana's *there you go*. This response does more than just confirm; it treats the correction as an accomplishment worthy of praise, essentially highlighting the breakdown even more. The offense seems to be restarted in lines 13 to 18, where Louise understandably attempts to account for her forgetfulness with *you know, I erased it. I don't like to remember* which Dana counters with *you can't erase everything, Mom*.

A similar antagonistic exchange occurs in the next excerpt (3.7) where Diane and Vera are walking through an antique store when Diane assesses an item on sale for Vera.

Here, after unsuccessful in getting Vera's reciprocated assessment, Diane admonishes Vera in line 12 by clarifying what Diane's original intent was not: *well, I don't want it*, meaning her talk did not communicate an intention to

```
3.7  $129.95
Vera, 11 December, 2003B

01  DIAN    Vera
02  VERA    ((Vera turns to Diane))
03  DIAN    look it- look it its only a hundred and twentynine,
04          ninetyfive
05  VERA    no but [we're going to go (for) [no
06  DIAN           [a::, -hu::ndre::d n        [twe::ntyni:::ne
07          ni:::netyfive
08  VERA    no wait. come on ((Vera starts to walk away; Diane
09          does not follow))
10          (1.0)
11          ((Vera turns around at beginning of lines 08 & 09))
12  DIAN    [well i don't (want) it
13  VERA    [wait-
14  VERA    wait til you go: were we go today.=
15  DIAN    =okay
```

buy the item. In doing so, Diane reacts to Vera's response for what it seems to lack in appreciation for her action. Similar to Dana's reaction above, we can presume that the co-participants' antagonistic responses are the result of their investment in the interaction (i.e., establishing the "correct" memory or securing a reciprocated assessment) and the patients' apparent disaffiliative response to that, but this assumes that the patients' actions were inherently offensive. The offense, it seems, is primarily a product of the interlocutor's actions. And while this offense is certainly predicated on the interlocutor's particular type of "investment," i.e., painful memory or aesthetic appreciation, it may also be a by-product of the interlocutors inability, due to the lack of other involved co-participants, to "retreat" interactionally from the course of action with the patient.

Fundamentally, though, the moral hostility is the product of the patient's co-participants. This can be seen by the excerpt below, which basically involves the same disruption that occurred in *Goatee*, ex. 04, but engenders a slightly more hostile reaction. Here, Jess and Dana are telling me about the local lake, when Louise abruptly asks me about the camera off to the side.

In line 24, after hearing Louise's "interruption," Dana sequences over Louise's utterances to the prior talk, similar to how she and I did in excerpt 04. Here though, Dana also raises her voice and glares at Louise. The disapproval, or moral hostility, that seems palpable here in this excerpt exists not only because of this change in Dana's voice quality and gaze, but because that then identifies the prior event at which we can perceive she is "angry" or frustrated. This suggests that the events potential for sanction, for instance, Louise's "interruptions" (for lack of a less evaluative term) in excerpts 04 and 08, are

```
    3.8 Camcorder
Louise, 10 September, 2003B

    14   JESS    I don't know whether that's
    15           you know, the kind of thing you like to do
    16           but it's really
    17           I mean <pretty::::,
    18           ((Dana does in-breath; Louise displays
    --           speaking next; Dana stops))
    19           [(during summer) it's gorgeous]
    20   LOIS    [is that thing going all the time?]
    --           ((pointing to camera; looking at Michael))
    21   MICH    yeah:,
    22           (1.0)
    23   LOIS    ((gives shoulder shrug))
    24   DANA    ((gazing at Louise)) <ITS AMAzing (.) how many
    25           people A::SK us> (0.2)[(0.2)=
    26   LOIS                          [huh?
    27   DANA    [=when we say we live in goldenlake villa
    28           [➤ ((looks to Michael))
```

what Goffman refers to as "virtual offenses" (1971, 108) meaning their moral assessment is not integral to their being interruptions but to someone treating them as such after the fact, suggesting that "morality" to a large degree is a retroactive affair.

My purpose here is not to suggest that the co-participants are "making it up" in the sense perceiving something that did not occur, or that FTD patients do not commit much greater offenses. These excerpts were selected first because they comprise the large majority of what occurs in daily life with the patients, and second because for more egregious offenses, there seems to be an inverse relation where the greater the breach is, the less people will acknowledge its occurrence. Analyzing these as disruptions or instances of FTD manifesting requires assuming then that they are transgressive in the first place. Notwithstanding these extreme cases, the data analyzed here suggests that if a moral deterioration in interaction with the patients does indeed occur, it does so through the progressive breakdown in the patients' ability to participate in sensible or coherent frameworks of action.

Insensibility, however, cannot fully explain how others perceive FTD, as patients are not simply seen as persons who act senselessly, but in some instances as persons who act in a "calculating" fashion, or childishly, or with prurient interests. Some sense of continuity or agency must then still be evident. Both Louise and Vera appeared to retain aspects of their former selves, such as well-preserved personal narratives, with Vera, of her financial endeavors, career, and family issues, and Louise, of her art training, career, and aptitude. In addition, both still seemed to maintain active interests as they did before, something that often troubled caregivers, such as Vera's continued attempts at managing her family's financial holdings. This ego-driven behavior is not always asocial. One notable example comes from a visit with Vera just prior to the Christmas holiday. Here, she showed little difficulty in her observance of either the holiday or in her obligations as a spouse, mother, or grandmother. She had extensively decorated her house and spent considerable time buying, organizing, and wrapping gifts for numerous family and friends. While she did receive help, Vera did not lack the motivation or procedural knowledge and selected age and gender appropriate gifts. Gift-giving is certainly prosocial but it also relates to a large part of Vera's autobiography as a wife, mother, and grandmother, and so relates to her maintenance as a certain person. The question then is how does this maintenance interact with the interactional 'insensibility' described above.

## Person-specific Bias

One insight into how this ego-maintenance plays out in social interaction may be found in Ing-Mari Tallberg's (1999) Swedish study on the semantic construction of *disdeictic confabulations* in FTD patients' responses to a semi-structured questionnaire. Her questions included current events as well as recent and distant events from the patients' autobiographical history. Tallberg discovered that the patients, in answering the questions, often altered the semantic content of the response even if that made the response patently wrong. The shifts occurred suddenly, without overt transitions or hesitation, but nevertheless were still treated by the patients as "answering the question." Most importantly, the shifts were strongly tilted to domains that were relevant to the identity of the patient, i.e., family and career, personal events, and persons, places, and things from one's memory, with deeper memories showing more recurrence (Tallberg 1999, 472). According to Tallberg, the patients' inability to provide the requested content threatened their *interactive identity* and, as compensation, their *identity-laden domains* projected unconsciously into their responses (Tallberg 1999, 476). Tallberg argued that this occurred because these memories are the ones "...most deeply connected to previously established cognitive and reactive patterns... [and are] closely related to the identity [of the patient] before the onset of disease" (Tallberg 1999, 474) and thus are relatively preserved and readily accessible.

Pragmatically, the fact that the patients' responses are confabulated is less important than their being produced as coherent answers, without attending to their possible, and sometimes evident, incongruence. This obliviousness suggests that the patients are largely *autonomous* for organizing their turns' construction (factual or otherwise) and do not orient to the relevance of others' prior or next actions. The prevalence of patients' responses being identity-laden is relevant when we consider that the allocation of turns, typed-actions, and speaker selection in the study was largely predetermined by the protocol. The intrusion of identity-laden responses was then seemingly spontaneous because of their probable conflict with the prior questions. And since the actions were analytically restricted to their performance as either questions or responses, what constituted *Identity* was necessarily determined by the response's versus the question's semantics. In naturally occurring talk, however, all of these aspects (speaker-selection, action-type, etc.) are determined organically by the co-participants' actions, and besides semantic content. Speakers have numerous channels besides semantics to project their identity: the production or omission of actions, action-types, and formulation, all of which are largely dependent on others' actions.

Nevertheless, a patient like the one described by Tallberg who had the same pattern of intrusive identity-laden responses, or person-specific talk, interacted with co-participants who were adaptive (unlike the tester in the protocol), this would result in a *Person-specific Bias* (PsB), whereby stability was better maintained when the patient's identity, or person, determined the talk's constitutive order. [3] Interactions may only require regulation, as seen through practices similar to those above, in those contexts where others' person-specific interests determined the courses of action. In the final analyses, two interactions will be presented in which both patients pursue similar courses of action that are equally relevant to their person-specific interests. As we will see, the stability of the interactions diverges radically, where one patient maintains her person-specific focus, while the other patient causes an unintended reversal in the central identity of the talk. In the first interaction below (Example 3/9a), Louise, her daughters, and I are driving back to their residence in silence, when Louise asks me, *do I act differently?*

Louise's question is notable, because it shows an awareness of her condition, which is not expected given FTD's association with lack of insight (see Chapter 1, Avineri, Chapter 5). Louise often showed awareness of her part in the ethnography, remarking that I should "write things down" when she forgot something, and sometimes became worried as to how she was perceived, so her question also serves as a means for determining the extent of these perceptions. The sequence from lines 01 to 08 is also notable, because Michael, through repetition, is evasively avoiding giving her an evaluation. Even when

---

3.   In utilizing terms like *autonomous, spontaneous,* or *person-specific bias* to describe the patients' talk or courses of action, the purpose is to specifically try and use descriptions that align with more mentalistic assessments typically attributed to FTD patients like *mental rigidity, perseveration, etc.*, without presupposing a corresponding argument about that mental phenomena. See also the discussion of the Rankin *et al.* (2008) paper in the Discussion section of this chapter.

```
3.9a Differently
Louise, 7 October, 2003D

((Family is traveling back home from going out to eat and going
shopping; After some silence, the interaction begins))
01   LOIS    <Do:: I: a:::ct> (2.0) differently?
02   MICH    Do you act differen[tly?
03   LOIS                       [Yeah
04   MICH    Then what?
05   LOIS    From the norm?
06   MICH    From the norm?
07   LOIS    Yeah
08   MICH    No, (.) not really
```

he does respond, evaluating Louise's behavior, *no, not really*, he mitigates it, not so much as to minimize its negative aspect ('no' in this case actually being the preferred response; see below), but rather, his certainty.

After this, Louise accounts for her questioning in lines 09 and 10 (Example 3.9b), to which Michael treats with the continuer *uh huh* in line 11 as not hearably complete. In line 13, she repeats her prior question in a expanded form, thus marking Michael's prior response as problematic and re-selecting him for a subsequent alternative. In lines 12, 14, and 15, Dana picks up on Louise's *frontotempera thing* and puns the word *tempera* (a type of paint) back to her mother loudly and while laughing. Also laughing, Louise replies back *well besides that!* After a small lull in the talk, Michael eventually does attempt to provide Louise with a more redeeming assessment in lines 20, 21, and 23, a response she seems to also treat as insufficient, as she only looks away while shaking her head. After a noticeable silence, Jess finally gives Louise a fuller and more authoritative assessment of her behavior, which Louise finally accepts (not shown).

In this excerpt, Louise displays a social competence that is remarkably different than previously expected of her by others (see Example 3.9c). For instance, her initial question, *do I act (2.0) differently* is given with a noticeable pause before the primary descriptor, displaying her difficulty in making this self-characterization. Her subsequent *from the norm* is more explicit as a relational description, but is also formatted from Michael's [differently] *then what?* When she does name her condition in *because I supposedly have this fronta tempura thing*, it is after another mitigation from Michael and before her more expanded repeat, *do I act any different from anybody else*, showing its engagement to still be in the service of securing a fuller response. Her word-choice in *supposedly* and *thing* shows a subtly dismissive stance towards the classification, especially for herself.

Procedurally, Louise's active interest in securing a self-assessment promotes her analytical acuity to the unfolding interaction—reducing her perceived autonomy—and accordingly affects a greater consequence on others, reducing the perceived spontaneity of her actions. In her initial talk with Michael,

```
3.9b Differently
Louise, 7 October, 2003D

09   LOIS    because I have I- I supposedly have fronta tempura
10           thing
11   MICH    uh huh,
12   DANA    tempura thing heh heh heh heh
13   LOIS    I- do I act any [different from anybody else?
14   DANA                   [it just gives you a very colorful
15           personality Ha hah hah hah hah
16   JESS    [(xxxx) tempura (xxx)-
17   LOIS    [well besides that::::::
18   MICH     [heh heh heh heh
19   LOIS     [heh heh heh heh heh
20   MICH    no. look it. that uh- that women that walked over,
21           that one that was complaining about the kids screaming
22   LOIS    yeah
23   MICH    yeah that was perfectly normal conversation
24           (P)
24   JESS    mom, you want to know how I think you act differently?
             (continued...)
```

the only autonomous and spontaneous action she produced was the initial question after the silence. After this, the autonomy of each action is invested in her interpretation of the prior action and consequently, none of her subsequent utterances can be described as spontaneous, or "surprising," to the unfolding interaction. As a result, she enforces others' accountability to her course of action both in the current sequence she is in, as well as events that may occur at its "periphery," for instance, in her picking up on Dana's laughing repeat. We can compare Louise's responsiveness here to excerpt 04, *Goatee,* in which her actions demonstrated almost a much greater autonomy from others' evident actions. Here, however, she is acutely responsive to the potential relevance of others' talk.

There is a socially awkward aspect to Louise's questioning. Her initial *do I act different* is designed to elicit a "yes" response (Raymond 2003), but doing so essentially confirms that she does act "differently." It then works like a self-deprecation, an action which prefers strong disagreement: "No, of course not!! You're perfectly fine!" (Pomerantz 1984, 92). The talk being person-specific should not be taken to mean that violations would be absent, but rather

```
3.9c Differently (formulations)

01   LOIS    <do:: I: a:::ct> (2.0) differently?
05   LOIS    from the norm?
09   LOIS    because I have I- I supposedly have Fronta tempura
10           thing
12   LOIS    I- do I act any [different from anybody else?
```

only that more stability would occur between the patient and co-participant actions.

The interaction below involving Vera shows the opposite trajectory where the person-specificity of the talk suddenly switches from Vera to another compromising her ability to function in what is essentially the same sequence but on an entirely different intersubjective "terrain." This excerpt is also relevant to the loss of socio-emotions in FTD, like empathy or concern for others (Hodges and Patterson 2007, 111). Before analyzing excerpt 3.12b, *Mother & Father*, it is necessary to first consider just her initial question (3.12a, below).

In the introductory section, I suggested that Vera seemed to lack concern for who I was or what my purposes were. It was then surprising later when analyzing the data to find questions like the ones below and see that Vera was indeed attempting to "situate me in her world" (Alessandro Duranti, personal communication). Looking at the other instances (and indeed the total number of occurrences), Vera did show concern, but one that was narrowly expressed. We can see this first with an extended interaction, where Vera, her other daughter Linda, her granddaughter Jane, and I are walking to lunch at a restaurant (occurrences are arrowed).

The next instance (Example 3.11, line 03) occurred during dinner with Vera, Bonnie, and I. This is the only time Vera asks my name, which occurred after we had met and after three hours into the visit.

Vera's questions all seem to act in determining the reason for the ethnographic visits. In excerpt 3.10, one can see an evolution of her question design from *where do you live* to the syntactically syncretic *how come you got here* to her final, *what are you doing here?* The last question is especially notable, because she produces it even before raising her head or having Michael's gaze, suggesting that this had been a question for which she was searching and had just occurred to her then. The question in excerpt 3.11, *Who are you with* is different because, like Louise's question, it orients to the institutional nature of the visits. In excerpt 3.12b, the question *where's your mother and father* works similarly, although by invoking a different relationship. Michael, however, treats it, simply as an unproblematic information-seeking question.

Like 3.9, in 3.12b, Michael initially avoids a response by repeating Vera's question, similar to the repairs in excerpt 06, lines 01–08 (Egbert 2004). Here, however, Vera simply confirms the question giving the floor back. After Michael's response in line 05, Bonnie begins *oh that's–* in lines 06, but

```
    3.12a Mother & Father
    Vera, 11 December, 2003D

    01  VERA    where's your mother and father?
```

```
3.10 What are you doing here?
Vera, 23 November 2003A

01              ((no current talk))
02  VERA➤  where do you LIve?
03          (2.0)
04  VERA➤  where do you live,
05  MICH    san delagado.
06          (0.8)
07  VERA    san delagado? (1.0) oh my god, where is that.
08          (0.6)
09  JANE    (really) far, honey,
10          (0.4)
11  VERA    I know. but where's San Delagado.
12  MICH    out towards the east
13  VERA    ºoh my godº
14          (3.0)
15  VERA    this is-                        ((looking down ))
16          (.)                      ((looks up to Michael ))
17          this is a wonder          ((points to ground ))
--          (50.0)                      ((still walking ))
19  VERA➤  so, how come you got here.   ((turns to Michael ))
20  MICH    huh,
21  VERA    how come you got here,
22  MICH    (why) am I out here?
23  VERA    yeah, you('re back) here.
24  MICH    how come I got here?
25  VERA    yeah.
26  MICH    I drove
--          (05min 45sec)   ((group now sitting in restaurant
--                           joined by Linda; Vera & Michael))
30  VERA    - ((gaze to Michael))       -
--  MICH    | ((gaze back & smiles))    |
--  VERA    | ((continues gaze))        |
--          |---------(1.8)---------- |
31  VERA    - ((gaze back down))        -
--          |---------(0.6)---------- |
32  VERA➤  |WHAt are| you doing here_
33          |--------|                 ((lifting gaze to Michael ))
34                   |--------------->   ((gaze on Michael ))
35  MICH    huh?
36  VERA    what are you doing here.
37  MICH    what am I doing [here=I'm doing a research study
38  VERA                    [ ((nods))
39  MICH    i'm doing a research study
40  VERA    a research [study?
41  MICH               [ ((nods))=
42  VERA    =o:::h ºhoney, (take) whatever you want,
43          eat whatever you want to eat ((offering to eat ))
            ((continued))
```

```
3.11 Who are you with?
Vera, 11 December 2003D

01              ((Prior talk between Bonnie & Michael))
02   VERA    now WAIt A minute,                 ((opens notebook))
03        ➤ what's your name.                   ((points to Michael))
04   MICH    |my name's (.) michael smith.
05   VERA    |---------------------- ➤ ((grabs & eats cookie ))
06           (1.6)
07   BONN    ºmichael
08           (4.8)                      ((Vera thumbs through pages))
09   VERA    m. i::, [(0.8)    ]c=h, a. e. l.      ((writing))
10   MICH           [º(mm mh)]      ((leans in, and lifts hand))
11   MICH    uh huh=
12   VERA    michael, smith.= [-      ((looks to Mich, then down))
13   MICH    mm mh           [-                   ((nods))
14           (1.8)                        ((Vera still writing))
15   VERA    |ºmm mh?
--          |--------|---        ➤ ((looks up expecting next ))
16   MICH    |  (1.0)  |---          ➤ ((does brow-flash ))
--                    |[mm?
17   VERA            [and who are you with?
18           (2.0)
19   MICH    put down doctor...        ((pointing to notebook))
--           ((text omitted))
20   VERA    and who is "michael smith",       (( " " reading))
21   MICH    me                         ((pointing to self))
```

is cut off by Vera's *passed away where?* Michael does not respond, and she self-repairs with *they died?* Her follow-up question (*how?*) is then produced with low volume and given with a lateral headshake, a combination that is often seen with assessments in stories, where speakers display an awed or unbelieving stance towards the event being assessed (M.H. Goodwin 1980; Schegloff 1987) This request-inform sequence occurs again, but when Vera inquires *well, how old were they* (line 16), Bonnie produces a noticeable brow-flash directed at Vera, showing surprise at Vera's continued questioning.

As Michael responds, Vera and Bonnie—in that order—both produce emphasized in-breaths in lines 18 and 19, a "response-cry" often associated with shock or dismay (Goffman 1981, 78). Vera also pulls back in an extended upright posture with an agape mouth and raised eyes, something that Bonnie also does. Describing the concurrent actions of both participants to this point, they initiate how an "empathic" reaction would appear publicly, and neither is less or more appropriate as such. Whether Vera's subjective experience supports empathy or its affective precursor is a separate issue from its practical appropriateness. At this point, Vera has produced actions that align with and often anticipate Bonnie's, and because the "normal" participant's actions mirror Vera's, this supports their appropriateness, while her surprise also marks them as unexpected.

In excerpt 3.12c, line 22, however, Vera states and *I'm seventy-two (.) and my husband is* as she toasts her co-participants with her common vocalizations *BIP* and *BOOP*. There is little that can be analyzed from Vera's TCUs: they are initiated on self-reference, are formatted on Michael's prior turn, and are celebrated by a toast. While seemingly unfitted to the prior course of action, she could be showing her thankfulness for her and her husband's longevity, which is not outside expectations. Its incongruity, however, can be inferred from the co-participants' laughter and them not treating Vera's utterances as actionable items, i.e., they did not return Vera's toast. The most situated measure of its destabilizing effect on the co-participants' prior talk appears at Bonnie's next question, *now what kind of cancer?* Here, she sequences back and over Vera's turns to Michael's earlier (lns 16, 20) turn and formulates the turn so as to maintain the prior order that existed before. Indeed, the *now* preface is often seen when speakers close an interceding activity to start the primary, and often shows the next talk to be part of "larger cumulative structure," which Vera's prior talk is actively being excluded from (Schiffrin 1988, 237). The turn-at-talk it picks up is also readably expandable, allowing Bonnie to address the reversal of person-specific talk and solve it by progressing the talk well past its prior inversion, which is continued through line 31. We even see her reprimand Michael and reference herself using an empathetic

```
    3.12b Mother & Father
    Vera, 11 December 2003D

    01   VERA    where's your mother and father?
    02   MICH    where's my- where's my mother and
    03           father?
    04   VERA    mm mh
    05   MICH    they passed away a few years ago
    06   BONN    oh that's [(xxx)-
    07   VERA              [passed away (where?)
    08           (1.0)
    09   VERA    they died?
    10   MICH    mm mh
    11           (2.0)
    12   VERA      ºhow,º ((shakes head))
    13   MICH    cancer
    14   BONN    [rea::^lly
    15   VERA    [well how old (were they)?
    16   BONN    ((does noticeable 'browflash' towards Vera))
    17   MICH    u:::::m my father was (.) fifty-five years old
    18   VERA    .HHHH      [HHHHHHH
    19   BONN               [.HHHHHHHHHH
    20   MICH    and my mother was fifty four
    21   BONN    oh my god
```

```
3.12c - Mother & Father
Vera, 11 December, 2003D

15   VERA    [well how old (were they)?
16   BONN    ((does noticeable 'browflash' towards Vera))
17   MICH    u:::::m my father was (.) fifty-five years old
18   VERA    .HHHH     [HHHHHHH
19   BONN              [.HHHHHHHHHH
20   MICH    and my mother was fifty four
21   BONN    oh my god
22   VERA    and I'm seventy two (.) and my husband is.
23   VERA    ((Lifts glass and toasts to Bonnie)) BI::::P
24   VERA    ((Toasts to Michael)) BOO::::P
25   BONN    heh heh [heh heh heh heh
26   MICH            [heh heh heh heh
27   BONN    now what kind of ca:::^cer?
28   MICH    ((text omitted))
29   BONN    ^and you still smoke?
30   BONN    I'll have to have the mother in me come out
31           and say <that is not a good thing>
32   BONN    because Vera's father- (.) her father died of
33           cancer(.) because he smoked and Vera gave it up
34   VERA    and I stopped smoking,
35   BONN    mm mh
36   VERA    I smoked smoked smoked.
```

membership-category with *I'm gonna have to have the mother in me come out and say that is not a good thing.*

After this, Bonnie now seems to prompt Vera's participation: *because Vera's father, her father died of cancer, because he smoked, and Vera gave it up.* This prompt is less successful compared to those analyzed before in facilitating Vera's response towards another co-participant, as her only responses are: *and I stopped smoking* and *I smoked smoked smoked,* both to Bonnie. Bonnie's attempt, however, is useful in showing the likely motivation for these practices as well as how specific they can be in supplying the necessary information for the patient. Bonnie's utterance is similar to what Harvey Sacks (Sacks and Jefferson 1995, 764) referred to as a *second story*, or a story given in response to a first story not only describing a similar situation but with the current and the prior storyteller in the same role. Sacks argued that in doing so, a speaker takes as their task to show that "one [current speaker] has listened [to the prior story] to be reminded of one's own experience and has understood the other's [prior storyteller's] experience" (Sacks and Jefferson 1995, 770). As such, second stories serve as a practical and useful means for exhibiting empathy to others. Bonnie, however, produces this second story with Vera's memories seeking not only to bring Vera into the interaction, but also to do so appositely with the current constitutive order. Overall, what seems un-empathic about Vera's actions was not a total absence of appropriate action, but rather a type of temporal failure in intersubjectivity whereby Vera is simply limited in maintaining the "empathic arc," or the progression of an order of events that matched others' presuppositions for normalcy, as predicated on another participant's prior disclosure, something Bonnie was able to see to its acceptable end.

## Discussion

The analysis from this study shows that the patients' co-participants use practices that have a similar agenda to those observed in Garfinkel's breaching tasks in which after the patients' breach, the co-participants either maintain the prior condition, (i.e., their interpretation and expectation for the current interaction) as the constitutive order or abandon it for a reconstituted order. This finding suggests that the moral feature attributed to FTD, while prevalent, may not indicate the loss of a particular moral faculty but may rather be a procedural or temporal artifact forced by decidedly more mundane infractions from the patients, and assessed morally by their interlocutors. Drawing on prior research (Tallberg 1999), it was suggested that interactional stability and normalcy are dependent on whether the patients or the co-participants' identity, or *person-specific courses of action*, organize the interaction: when constituted by the patient's, not only are the compensatory caregiver practices absent, but there is greater stability to the interlocutors' concerted actions. In contrast, when the talk is organized by another co-participant, we see compensatory practices deployed and (assume) less stability to concerted action. This is most evident in the final analyses where perturbations in the stability of the interaction only arise when the prevailing course of action separates from the patient's person-specific interests.

In the introduction of this chapter, it was argued that the moral assessment of FTD patients' abnormal behavior, though endemic, is descriptively and categorically problematic. Garfinkel's procedural model of morality suggests why this is: the moral assessment of an infraction is determined *post hoc* to the actual appearance of the infraction, and thus is not a necessary attribute of the behavior. Likewise, this should caution us against simply applying (im)moral attributes to the neuroanatomical deficits suspected, as the moral assessment is only fully constituted in others' phenomenological apperception. It should not, however, stop the exploration of its origins; moral attributions like transgression, misconduct, and inappropriateness are not only an important part of caregivers' reports in FTD, but are an integral part to what makes us human.

One framework—the preference of the patient's person-specific interests over others—does seem to be more intrinsically moral as it would affect the patients' attending to others' intentions and empathizing with others feelings, and presumably would be what engender others' assessments of FTD patients being "selfish," "self-absorbed," or "indifferent to others" (Miller *et al.* 1997; Neary *et al.* 1998). This should not be taken to mean that this person-specificity will only serve selfish, asocial interests however. Not only does something like Vera's gift-giving undermine this interpretation but many infractions, though inappropriately placed, could not so easily take this assessment. In Tallberg's study, this was attributed to the selective preservation of identity-laden domains in the patients' cognition or underlying neurological structures. The tendency for patients and others to rely on person-specific courses of action may then be because these are the only ones remaining where the patients have enough sufficiently retained experience to coordinate perception and action. Some studies have found FTD patients to be markedly less competent than controls or Alzheimer patients in theory of mind, social cognition, or making social inferences (Gregory *et al.* 2002; Kipps and Hodges 2006; Kipps *et al.* 2009; Lough and Hodges, 2002). Such a view could be complementary to this chapter's behavioral description as without insight into or concern for what others' courses of action may suggest about their intentions for interests, the patients would be unable to build concerted action.

At a behavioral level though, whatever the neurobiological bases, FTD's behavioral disorder, if it can be said to manifest in interaction, does so *temporally*, meaning the patients do not do what is expected of them *at the moment it is expected*. Behaviorally, this should compel us to look not only at the nature of the patients' (in)actions but also their temporal placement prior to and after others' actions. A recent study has suggested that such an interest would even have clinical implications. In Rankin *et al.* (2008), building off the model of FTD as "acquired sociopathy," used a forensics psychometric and found that behavioral variant FTD and semantic dementia patients, compared to both normals and other dementias, produced more "spontaneous social behaviors" such as in perseverating on "1 to 2 pet topics" during the examination disallowing the "...clinical interaction to proceed fluidly," repeatedly interrupting the medical examinations, "...spoke in a tangential, rambling manner that shifted to irrelevant topics...[and derail]...the course of the clinical interaction" (69–70). As the analysis in this chapter has suggested, however, characterizations such as "spontaeneous," "perseveration," "interruption," "tangential," "irrelevant topics," etc., are not given simply because they are so, but because they are determined by the co-participants' concerted action as determined by the interactional order given for a clinical encounter to which they themselves adhere. Most succinctly, their expectations for a certain temporal order and placement of actions define the non-normative placement of the FTD patients' actions.

The prevalence of moral attribution supports the use of instruments specifically designed for eliciting caregivers' assessments of the patient through inventories or personal and interpersonal scales in identifying FTD. This study cautions, however, that while these instruments do differentiate FTD from other dementias, they also reflect a perception that may lead caregivers to alternative explanations for the patients' behavioral changes, explanations that are decidedly more prejudiced in nature, leading to delays in seeking medical consult, and possibly to estrangement. Though to best knowledge, no study known of investigates whether lay perceptions delay diagnosis, or the rate at which patients lose social relations prior to diagnosis as opposed to after, this can be inferred from multiple sources: the presence of patient and family estrangement in case histories (Cox 2007, 37–38; Faber *et al.* 2003; Graham 2007. Mourik *et al.* 2004), the findings of the Ibach *et al.*, study (2003), where out of 33 patients found with FTD in psychiatric hospitals, only one had been diagnosed prior to institutionalization (c.f. Chapter 1, Introduction, epidemiology, this volume), the tendency of physicians and caregivers to misperceive early alterations as having other causes (Dell and Halford 2002; Rankin *et al.* 2008, 69), and the difficulty that caregivers often have in not reacting angrily towards the patients after diagnosis (Lough and Garfoot 2007, 302). As such, one fear among clinical workers is that FTD patients, more the behavioral variant, are never recognized by family, friends, or clinicians as having a neuro-degenerative illness, and instead are institutionalized or "...live as deteriorating, treatment-resistant social recluses [or exiles]" (Rankin *et al.* 2008, 69).

One reason this may be the case has to do with what is in fact a by-product of moral assessment, but plays an integral factor in interpersonal relations: personal responsibility. Erving Goffman argued that moral sanctions and rewards were only effective insofar as they defined the actor's responsibility in either being unaware, negligent, knowing of, or with the full intention of the consequences of his or her actions (1971, 98). Others not only attended to his or her acts being potentially violative, but also to his or her orienting to this, and then being apologetic or making amends afterwards, two orientations that FTD patients, because of their limitations, would not likely do, which according to Goffman could "...reflect more harshly on them than does the original offense" (100). Rather than appearing specifically as a *lack of ability*, as presumably Alzheimer and aphasia patients would because of their own perception; FTD may appear to others primarily as a *lack of willingness* whereby they lack the moral constitution to enact moral, or resist immoral, actions. Consideration of these facts and possibilities then make it imperative that we move past classifications of behavior to their actual description *in situ*.

## Conclusion

Though this current study's analysis, being primarily descriptive, is limited in being fully answerable to neuro-psychiatric concerns, its ability to provide a socio-behavioral description of FTD is argued to be its most important contribution. If, as argued by some, it is better to classify or focus on FTD as a behavioral as opposed to cognitive dementia (Pijnenburg *et al.* 2004; Rankin *et al.* 2008), it is essential for researchers to fully explore its behavioral manifestation, as it is its neuro-anatomical underpinnings. The explicit premise in conversation analysis is that social interaction is not unorganized or random but is highly structured, recurrent, and is both independent and dependent on the coordinated engagement of its users (Sacks *et al.* 1974). Our most current models of the structure and organization of interaction are then relevant to the models developed for understanding how FTD manifests, and the brain functions, in social interaction. While problematic for neurological analysis, this organization is rendered empirically observable through interactional analysis and from there, recurrent organizations can be identified, given formal description—as they in many cases have been—and then be applied "inward" to a description of how brains in concert maintain that social organization. This is in essence what "reverse-engineering," the process endorsed in the title of this volume, describes, and what Harvey Sacks presciently advocated in his early lecture, *The Inference-Making Machine* where he argues that our responsibility as interactional researchers is to not let our notions of the "complexity or simplicity of the apparatus" (the brain) or the "face-value complexity or simplicity of the object" (the action or event) determine what must be occurring, but rather focus solely on the objects of interaction and from there 'build the brains' these objects required (Sacks and Jefferson 1995, 115). Fully reverse engineering the social brain then will not only explain its design and function through psychometric tasks, but ultimately in reference to the social practices, obligations, and consequences that humans—as members of a society—face in everyday existence.

## References

Bolden, G.B.

2006  Little Words That Matter: Discourse Markers "So" and "Oh" and the Doing of Other-Attentiveness in Social Interaction. *Journal of Communication* 56(4): 661–688.

Bozeat, S., C.A. Gregory, M.A.L. Ralph and J.R. Hodges.

2000  Which neuropsychiatric and behavioural features distinguish frontal and temporal variants of frontotemporal dementia from Alzheimer's disease? *J Neurol Neurosurg Psychiatry* 69(2): 178–186.

Cox, C.B.

2007  *Dementia and social work practice: research and interventions.* New York: Springer.

Dell, D.L. and J.J. Halford.

2002  Dementia presenting as postpartum depression. *Obstetrics and Gynecology* 99(5,2): 925–928.

Egbert, M.

2004  Other-initiated repair and membership categorization—some conversational events that trigger linguistic and regional membership categorization. *Journal of Pragmatics* 36(8): 1467–1498.

Faber, R., V.M. Hill and B.J. Kim.

2003  Frontotemporal dementia affecting a U.S. Air Force officer. *Military Medicine* 168(4): 333–336.

Garfinkel, H.

1963  A Conception of, and Experiments with 'Trust' as a Condition of Stable Concerted Actions. In *Motivation and Social Interaction,* edited by O.J. Harvey, 187–238. New York: Ronald Press.

Goffman, E.

1971  *Relations in Public: Microstudies of the Public Order.* New York: Basic Books.

1972  *Relations in public: Microstudies of the public order.* New York: Harper and Row.

1981  *Forms of talk.* University of Pennsylvania publications in conduct and communication. Philadelphia: University of Pennsylvania Press.

Goodwin, C.

1986  Audience Diversity, Participation and Interpretation. *Text* 6(3): 283–316.

2003  Recognizing Assessable Names. In *Studies in language and social interaction,* edited by P.J. Glenn, C.D. LeBaron, J.S. Mandelbaum and R. Hopper, 128–136. LEA communication series. Mahwah, NJ: Erlbaum.

2007  Participation, Stance, and Affect in the Organization of Activities. *Discourse and Society,* 18(1): 53–73.

Goodwin, C. and M.H. Goodwin.

1992  Assessments and the construction of context. In *Rethinking Context: Language as an Interactive Phenomenon,* edited by A. Duranti and C. Goodwin, 147–190. Studies in the Social and Cultural Foundations of Language. Cambridge: Cambridge University Press.

Goodwin, M.H.

1980 Processes of Mutual Monitoring Implicated in the Production of Description Sequences. *Sociological Inquiry* 50(3–4): 303–317.

1990 *He-said-she-said : talk as social organization among Black children*. Bloomington: Indiana University Press.

Graham, A.

2007 Epidemiology of frontotemporal dementia. In *Frontotemporal Dementia Syndromes*, edited by J.R. Hodges, 25-37. Cambridge: Cambridge University Press.

Gregory, C., S. Lough, V. Stone, S. Erzinclioglu, L. Martin, S. Baron-Cohen and J.R. Hodges.

2002 Theory of mind in patients with frontal variant frontotemporal dementia and Alzheimer's disease: theoretical and practical implications. *Brain: A Journal of Neurology* 125(4): 752–764.

Heritage, J.

1984a *Garfinkel and ethnomethodology*. Cambridge: Polity Press.

1984b *A Change of State Token and Aspects of its Sequential Placement*. Studies in emotion and social interaction. Edited by J.M. Atkinson and J. Heritage. Cambridge: Cambridge University Press; Paris: Editions de la Maison des sciences de l'homme.

2002 Oh-prefaced responses to assessments: a method of modifying agreement/disagreement. In *The language of turn and sequence*, edited by C.E. Ford, B.A. Fox and S.A. Thompson, 196–224. Oxford studies in sociolinguistics. Oxford: Oxford University Press.

Heritage, J. and G. Raymond.

2005 The Terms of Agreement: Indexing Epistemic Authority and Subordination in Talk-in-Interaction. *Social Psychology Quarterly* 68(1): 15–38.

Hodges, J.R. and K. Patterson.

2007 The Neuropsychology of Frontotemporal Dementia. In *Frontotemporal Dementia Syndromes*, edited by J.R. Hodges, 102–133. Cambridge: Cambridge University Press.

Hutchby, I. and R. Wooffitt.

1998 *Conversation analysis : principles, practices, and applications*. Cambridge: Polity Press.

Ibach B, H. Koch, M Koller, M Wolfersdorf.

2003   Hospital admission circumstances and prevalence of frontotemporal lobar degeneration: a multicenter psychiatric state hospital study in Germany. *Dementia and Geriatric Cognitive Disorders* 16(4): 253–264.

Jefferson, G.

1991   List Construction as a Task and Resource. In *Interactional Competence,* edited by G. Psathas, 63–92. New York: Irvington Publishers.

Jung, R. and K. Solomon.

1993   Clinical Practice and Service Development: Psychiatric Manifestations of Pick's Disease. *International Psychogeriatrics* 5(2): 187–202.

Kipps, C.M., P.J. Nestor, J. Acosta-Cabronero, R. Arnold and J.R. Hodges.

2009   Understanding social dysfunction in the behavioural variant of frontotemporal dementia: the role of emotion and sarcasm processing. *Brain: A Journal of Neurology* 132(3): 592–603.

Kipps, C.M. and J.R. Hodges.

2006   Theory of mind in frontotemporal dementia. *Social Neuroscience* 1(3–4): 235–244.

Levinson, S.C.

2000   *Pragmatics*. Cambridge: Cambridge University Press.

Lough, S. and V. Garfoot.

2007   Psychological interventions in frontotemporal dementia. In *Frontotemporal Dementia Syndromes,* edited by J.R. Hodges, 277–325. Cambridge: Cambridge University Press.

Lough, S. and J.R. Hodges.

2002   Measuring and modifying abnormal social cognition in frontal variant frontotemporal dementia. *Journal of Psychosomatic Research* 53(2): 639–646.

Mendez, M.F.

2006   What frontotemporal dementia reveals about the neurobiological basis of morality. *Medical Hypotheses* 67(2): 411–418.

Mendez, M.F., E. Anderson and J.S. Shapira

2005   An investigation of moral judgement in frontotemporal dementia. *Cognitive and Behavioral Neurology: Official Journal of the Society for Behavioral and Cognitive Neurology* 18(4): 193–197.

Mendez, M.F., A.K. Chen, J.S.Shapira, P. Lu and B.L. Miller.

2006 Acquired extroversion associated with bitemporal variant of frontotemporal dementia. *The Journal of Neuropsychiatry and Clinical Neurosciences*, 18(1): 100–107.

Mendez, M.F., A.K. Chen, J.S. Shapira and B.L. Miller.

2005 Acquired sociopathy and frontotemporal dementia. *Dementia and Geriatric Cognitive Disorders* 20(2–3): 99–104.

Miller, B., A. Darby, D. Benson, J. Cummings and M. Miller.

1997 Aggressive, socially disruptive and antisocial behaviour associated with fronto-temporal dementia. *British Journal of Psychiatry* 170(FEB.): 150–155.

Mourik, J.C., S.M.Rosso, M.F. Niermeijer, H.J. Duivenvoorden, J.C. Van Swieten and A. Tibben.

2004 Frontotemporal dementia: behavioral symptoms and caregiver distress. *Dementia and Geriatric Cognitive Disorders* 18(3–4): 299–306.

Mychack, P., H. Rosen and B.L. Miller.

2001 Novel Applications of Social-Personality Measures to the Study of Dementia. *Neurocase: The Neural Basis of Cognition* 7(2): 131–143.

Neary, D., J.S. Snowden, L. Gustafson, U. Passant, D. Stuss, S. Black, M. Freedman, A. Kertesz, P.H. Robert, M. Albert, K. Boone, B.L. Miller, J. Cummings and D.F. Benson.

1998 Frontotemporal lobar degeneration: A consensus on clinical diagnostic criteria. *Neurology* 51(6): 1546–1554.

Pijnenburg, Y.A.L., F. Gillissen, C. Jonker and P. Scheltens.

2004 Initial complaints in frontotemporal lobar degeneration. *Dementia and Geriatric Cognitive Disorders* 17(4): 302–306.

Pomerantz, A.

1984 Agreeing and disagreeing with assessments: Some features of preferred/dispreferred turn shapes. In *Structures of social action : studies in conversation analysis,* edited by J.M. Atkinson and J. Heritage, 57–101. Cambridge: Cambridge University Press.

Potter, J.

2005 Making psychology relevant. *Discourse Society* 16(5): 739–747.

Rankin, K.P., E. Baldwin, C. Pace-Savitsky, J.H. Kramer and B.L. Miller.

2005 Self awareness and personality change in dementia. *J Neurol Neurosurg Psy-*

chiatry 76(5): 632–639.

Rankin, K.P., J.H. Kramer and B.L. Miller.

2005   Patterns of cognitive and emotional empathy in frontotemporal lobar degeneration. *Cognitive and Behavioral Neurology: Official Journal of the Society for Behavioral and Cognitive Neurology* 18(1): 28–36.

Rankin, K.P., H.J. Rosen, J.H. Kramer, G.F. Schauer, M.W. Weiner, N. Schuff, and B.L. Miller.

2004   Right and left medial orbitofrontal volumes show an opposite relationship to agreeableness in FTD. *Dementia and Geriatric Cognitive Disorders* 17(4): 328–332.

Rankin, K.P., W. Santos-Modesitt, J.H. Kramer, D. Pavlic, V. Beckman and B.L. Miller.

2008   Spontaneous social behaviors discriminate behavioral dementias from psychiatric disorders and other dementias. *The Journal of Clinical Psychiatry* 69(1): 60–73.

Rankin, K.P., J.H. Kramer, P. Mychack, B.L. Miller.

2003   Double dissociation of social functioning in frontotemporal dementia. *Neurology* 60(2): 266–271.

Raymond, G.

2003   Grammar and Social Organization: Yes/No Interrogatives and the Structure of Responding. *American Sociological Review* 68(6): 939–967.

Raymond, G. and J. Heritage.

2006   The Epistemics of Social Relations: Owning Grandchildren. *Language in Society* 35(05): 677–705

Sacks, H.

1967   'The Search For Help: No One To Turn To.' In Essays in SelfDELETE Destruction, edited by E.S. Shneidman, 203–223. New York: Science House.

Sacks, H., E.A. Schegloff and G. Jefferson.

1974   A Simplest Systematics for the Organization of Turn-Taking for Conversation. *Language* 50(4): 696–735

Sacks, H. and G. Jefferson.

1995   *Lectures on conversation.* Oxford: Blackwell.

Schegloff, E.A.

1987 Analyzing Single Episodes of Interaction: An Exercise in Conversation Analysis. *Social Psychology Quarterly* 50(2): 101–114.

2007 *Sequence organization in interaction : a primer in conversation analysis I*. Cambridge: Cambridge University Press.

Schegloff, E.A. and H. Sacks.

1973 Opening Up Closings. *Semiotica* 8(4): 289–327.

Schiffrin, D.

1988 *Discourse markers*. Studies in interactional sociolinguistics, vol 5. Cambridge: Cambridge University Press.

Selting, M.

2007 Lists as embedded structures and the prosody of list construction as an interactional resource. *Journal of Pragmatics* 39(3): 483–526

Tallberg, I.

1999 Projection of Meaning in Fronto-Temporal Dementia. *Discourse Studies* 1(4): 455–477.

$$— 4 —$$

# Examining Perseverative Behaviors of a Fronto-temporal Dementia Patient and Caregiver Responses: The Benefits of Observing Ordinary Interactions and Reflections on Caregiver Stress


Lisa Mikesell


Unlike most dementias, which are defined by a decline in *cognitive* functioning (Molloy and Lubinski 1991), frontotemporal dementia (FTD) shows a change and decline in *social* competence. (In)competence, whether cognitive or social, is defined by clinicians or those with the authority to designate a given behavior as deviant or pathological (see Harding and Palfrey 1997). Clinical assessments of FTD incompetence typically begin with observations of FTD patients during clinical interviews and neuropsychological testing. These interactions are typically brief, infrequent, and structured. To get a fuller picture of FTD patients' behaviors, clinicians' also rely on the behaviors that are reported by caregivers. Caregivers' perceptions of socially inappropriate behavior are thus an important piece in the diagnostic process. Caregivers' reports, although not based on brief or limited experiences with patients like clinical reports, may be problematic because they are filtered through memory. Additionally, some types of behaviors may be difficult to articulate or may be perceived as less challenging to manage and may thus go unreported. To supplement clinicians' assessments from structured interviews and caregivers' secondhand reports, this chapter, in the tradition of ethnomethodology (see Heritage 1984b for a review and history of ethnomethodology; see Maynard and Clayman 1991 for a review of ethnomethodology and its relationship to conversation analysis), relies on direct observations of everyday interactions to explore the behaviors of FTD patients and caregiver responses in natural social settings. More specifically, this chapter (as do others in this volume) applies conversation analysis (CA), which requires audio- and/or video-recordings of naturally occurring interactions. Heritage and Atkinson (1984, 2–3) explain how such an insistence on the use of recordings differs from other research traditions and, in doing so, outline why CA is particularly useful for understanding FTD social behavior. They state,

> [m]ost obviously, [conversation analysis] represents a departure both from the use of interviewing techniques in which the verbal reports of interview subjects are treated as acceptable surrogates for the observation of actual behavior and from the use of experimental methodologies in which the social scientist must necessarily manipulate, direct, or otherwise intervene in the subjects' behavior. It also contrasts with observational studies in which data are recorded in field notes or with the use of precoded schedules.

A thorough understanding of FTD behavior is clinically important because FTD is diagnosed based on clusters of behaviors (see Appendix A for the FTD diagnostic criteria, Neary *et al.* 1998). Structural and functional imaging, for instance, are no guarantee for an accurate diagnosis of any dementia (Osimani and Freedman 1991, 22) including FTD (Mendez *et al.* 2005, 4). As a result, diagnosis requires an accurate description of FTD behaviors. FTD behaviors have, of course, been characterized as socially incompetent. Patients have been reported to demonstrate impaired tactfulness and manners, violations of interpersonal space, inappropriate touching, overt sexual behavior, impulsivity, and verbal and physical disinhibition (Jagust *et al.* 1989). They have also been reported to lack sympathy, empathy, emotional warmth, embarrassment, and awareness of the needs of others (Miller *et al.* 2001). While few would argue that these behaviors do not constitute social incompetence, social inappropriateness is most clearly defined *interactionally* and in ordinary social contexts, which is also where family and friends first notice and experience a patient's behaviors. To examine the social deficits of FTD patients, we must ask what such behaviors look like in everyday interactions and examine how other participants respond to these behaviors in social contexts.

Examining "ordinary" interactions between FTD patients and other interlocutors helps elucidate the nature and range of FTD behaviors in social interactions and the kinds of management practices caregivers use as well as their effectiveness. Examining these management practices in turn provides a unique window into caregivers' daily routines, particularly the responsibilities they take on to both manage inappropriate behavior of patients and to maintain or restore the order of the interaction. This chapter, therefore, has several aims: One aim is to explore the nature of a patient's inappropriate behaviors in interaction, focusing on perseverative behaviors (i.e., the "repetition of ideas" or "information redundancy" [Ulatowska and Chapman 1991, 115]) which is one of the diagnostic criteria for FTD (see Appendix A). What can we learn from direct observations of inappropriate and perseverative behaviors that was not already known from caregivers' reports and clinical interviews? What does it mean, in a practical sense, to show a "decline in social interpersonal conduct" (a core diagnostic feature), "distractibility and impersistence" or "perseverative and stereotyped behaviour" (supportive diagnostic features, Neary *et al.* 1998, see Appendix A)? A close look at contextualized perseverative behaviors helps address these questions. A second aim is to document how caregivers attempt to manage inappropriate behaviors and how such attempts influence the interaction. How do caregiver responses (attempt to) preserve or restructure the interaction? What do their responses reveal about how the perseverative behaviors disrupt the interactional structure in the first place? In other words, what are the structures of interaction that caregivers perceive to be important to preserve? A third aim is to consider the nature and extent of the responsibilities taken on by caregivers and other interlocutors when FTD patients do not adhere to social expectations, and how these responsibilities may contribute to the stress of being an FTD caregiver.

To meet these aims, this chapter examines how caregivers and other interactants manage the perseverative behaviors of an individual diagnosed with FTD during everyday interactions. The examination of ordinary interactions requires the use of audio and videotaped footage of natural and spontaneous interactions between FTD patients and their interlocutors. Interlocutors do not treat all the behaviors of the patient as inappropriate; thus, this analysis carefully considers those behaviors that *are* treated as inappropriate, recognizing that interlocutors are likely to address those that are particularly interruptive to the ongoing collaborative project or goals of the participants and therefore those that are most socially disruptive. Given that "there is little to guide clinicians in terms of assessing and managing problems for sufferers, carers and family members" (Lough and Garfoot 2007, 285), this approach to FTD provides a unique perspective, one that may be helpful for both caregivers and clinicians facing practical, real-world considerations.

The first section of the chapter discusses caregiver reports of FTD behaviors and argues for the need to examine behaviors in ordinary interactions and through direct observation. The second section focuses on audio and/or video recorded FTD behaviors, specifically "perseverative and stereotyped behaviours" (Neary *et al.* 1998, see Appendix A), and how interlocutors manage, that is interrupt or stop, the perseverative behaviors they deem to be inappropriate. This section highlights two common practices interlocutors employ to deal with such perseverative behaviors as well as the patient's responses to these management attempts: the first practice involves reasoning or explaining a more appropriate or less disruptive behavior than the current behavior, while the second practice attempts to intervene in the ongoing perseverative behavior by distracting the patient. It is, of course, the interlocutors' attempts to manage or control the perseverative behaviors that illuminate what the problem is, that is, the aspect or feature of the behavior that is being addressed or sanctioned and thus treated as inappropriate. The third section documents a third practice interlocutors use to manage FTD behavior. When the social context does not allow caregivers to focus explicitly on the patient, caregivers are unable to address the behavior using discourse practices (i.e., talk). Instead, caregivers often opt to use physical guidance or prompting. After discussing the nature of such inappropriate behaviors in ordinary interaction and how interlocutors attempt to manage them, the last section reflects on what we have learned from direct observations of these behaviors including how such an investigation illuminates the burden placed on caregivers during 'ordinary' interaction and how these seemingly small social moments are likely considerable sources of caregiver stress.

## The Data, Participants, and Perseveration

This analysis focuses primarily on Kelly, who was introduced by Torrisi in Chapter 2 of this volume. Kelly's changes became noticeable to her husband in 2003. She was diagnosed with semantic dementia and FTD in 2005. Torrisi outlined the nature of Kelly's perseverative behaviors, noting that they tend to be complex in nature (i.e., require multiple steps to accomplish), something which will become clear in the extracts below. The other participants in the data include Kelly's husband, Bron; the ethnographer, Sam, who visited Kelly over the course of ten months (from December 4, 2006 to October 10, 2007) and collected seven hours of audio and/or video of ordinary interactions and nearly five hours of caregiver interviews; Elinor, the owner and head nurse of the care facility where Kelly had been staying for seven weeks before this video data was collected; and two facility staff members: Rachel and Gina.

### Caregiver testimonies and the importance of observing ordinary interactions

This section briefly discusses caregivers' (usually spouses') stories, from both doctors' notes and from interviews with caregivers. Caregivers' reports of behavioral changes in FTD are particularly important because, as mentioned above, diagnosis relies on behavioral criteria, much of which is documented through caregivers' descriptions of patients' behaviors. While these second-hand reports range in content, often caregiver testimonies reveal particularly striking or extreme behaviors. During a single FTD consensus meeting, where doctors and clinicians discuss diagnosis and patient updates, several caregivers' testimonies were reported, and included the following incidents and behaviors: a father throwing up on a plate at dinner and passing it to his children, unusual and excessive hording behavior and compulsive spending on selected items such as condiments, decreased personal hygiene, and irrational, angry outbursts (Mikesell, April 19, 2006: field notes). Caregivers' reports of extreme behaviors may be due to the difficulty they experience in receiving an accurate diagnosis. Sometimes caregivers' stories are doubted in the early stages of the dementia. As a result, diagnosis can be delayed even as the patient's behaviors become more extreme. Following an early doctor's visit, the wife of one of the FTD patients in our ethnographic study received the following report of her husband: "although he was able to give a detailed history of his life to date, his wife would anxiously fill in any gaps she felt his story was missing." The frustration that caregivers experience with the diagnostic process may eventually cause them to report extreme behaviors early during doctors' visits, so as to make clear the gravity of the situation that may not always be visible in the clinic.

Interviews with caregivers have also revealed extreme inappropriate behaviors. UCSF, where one of the leading clinics treating FTD is located, began producing a documentary to raise public awareness of FTD. In the video-recorded interviews three women describe the behaviors of their husbands who have been diagnosed with FTD (from http://www.memory.ucsf.edu/Documentary_Site/film.html):

A.  He will go outside and set on the ground for two hours and kill ants. And he lets them crawl up on his hand an' then 'e picks 'em off an' puts 'em in a bucket and counts 'em and he keeps track of it an' he'll come in and write down that he's killed 985 ants, today; an' he does our neighbors yard too and tells our neighbor how many ants he's killed.

B.  He would bike to work and um change in his cubicle? you know? Not the bathroom. *((smile voice))* 'n m Nick. *((reported speech displaying embarrassment and concern))*

C.  He pulled my daughter who wasn't wearing a lifejacket and didn't have 'er inner tube; he p- took a stick and they were playing a game and he pulled her out into the deep part of the river where the current was fast and then he dropped the stick an' swam away.

A and B's reports tell of recurring behaviors that are unusual, one compulsive, the other breaking strong social mores, while C reports a single incident that was particularly worrisome and consequential to the lives of their family. In my own interviews with caregivers, similar extreme behaviors are often reported early on in the interview process. Io, the primary caretaker of Juno, a 65-year old woman diagnosed with FTD approximately two years earlier, revealed that Juno often refused to shower and would call people at all hours of the night for mundane reasons (Mikesell, November, 30, 2006: field notes). Similarly, when Kelly was moved to her current facility, a staff member reported that she went to the bathroom in a waste basket in her room and aggressively pinched one of the staff's nipples. These reports and interviews document behaviors that are clearly disruptive to the daily lives and social relationships of these patients and their families, and they are likely a reason why caring for FTD patients is perhaps more difficult and stressful than caring for people with other dementias (Lough and Garfoot 2007).

These behaviors reported in stories seem to be most salient to the caregivers and other loved ones. It is thus important to document ways in which caregivers attempt to manage extreme behaviors such as the ones commonly reported in caregiver interviews. Io reported that when Juno became aggressive and grabbed her, Io would hold Juno's wrists, look her in the eye, and say to her *I'm your friend. I'm nice to you. You should be nice to me.* Io also reported that she removed all the knives from the kitchen to prevent any mishaps and began locking her door at night (Mikesell, November 30, 2006: field notes). A look at the range of caregiver strategies shows they consist of direct management tactics that try to alter the patient's behavior in progress or the patient's understanding of a situation as well as those that are preventative.

There are also management practices that address behaviors that are not as extreme, but that involve moments that occur in ordinary discourse. Indeed, it is likely that the incremental building up of small transgressions is as great a strain on the relationships between caregivers and patients as are the extreme social deviances. These behaviors and management practices are equally important to document and analyze, because, in contrast to many of the reported extreme behaviors and some diagnostic criteria, these behaviors may be more amenable to direct observation in the clinic where diagnosis begins.

## Managing Perseveration

The following excerpts focus primarily on Kelly. As will become evident in the interactions presented, her semantic dementia does not appear to be particularly problematic in ordinary interactions; she does, however, frequently demonstrate behaviors included in the consensus guidelines for the diagnosis of FTD, predominantly in the "speech and language" category: "stereotypy of speech and perseveration," and in the "behavioural disorder" category: "perseverative and stereotyped behaviour" (see Appendix A for consensus guidelines, Neary *et al.* 1998). As she had been moved to a facility on a trial basis several weeks earlier, these recordings are from a relatively new environment and a new routine. Kelly, until recently, was a piano teacher, and before moving to the facility her perseverative behavior and talk concerned when her students' appointments were scheduled. In her new environment, she fixates primarily on two activities: using the phone and checking her medication. The excerpts below illustrate her perseverative behaviors in ordinary interactions and focus on interactions in which her interlocutors treat these behaviors as inappropriate and disruptive. As such, the analysis presented also highlights the ways in which her interlocutors attempt to manage her perseverative behaviors.

### *Reasoning and explaining*

Example 4.1[1] shows Kelly looking at a chart in her room that indicates the times she must take her medication as well as the doses of medication she has already taken. Because Kelly constantly checks her medicine and whether she took it, one of the staff members and Kelly's husband, Bron, suggested that she keep a second, portable chart in her purse. Nevertheless, Kelly insists on checking the chart in her room. In Example 4.1, Kelly's interlocutor, Sam, reminds Kelly to check the chart in her bag instead and tries to get her accustomed to using it. (Please see Appendix B for transcription notations.)

In line 9, Sam attempts to explain why she can use the one in her bag, telling her the chart is the same as the one in her room. In lines 22–24, 26, Sam elaborates further, explaining that there is a benefit to using the one in her bag: she does not have to get up all the time. In lines 13, 15, 17, and 19, Kelly aligns with Sam and agrees that both charts are the same. Furthermore, in lines 27 and 31, she shows that she understands how Sam's suggestion is useful by offering her own formulation of the benefit Sam articulates in lines 24 and 26. Yet, despite Kelly's *displays* of understanding, she never *demonstrates* such understanding: She continues to check the chart in her room rather than the one in her bag. Indeed, in Example 4.2 below, approximately two minutes after Example 4.1, Sam again tries to interrupt Kelly's behavior and stop her from using the chart in her room.

In line 7 of example 4.2, Sam tells Kelly to check her bag for the chart rather than use the chart on her desk. In lines 14, 16, 19, and 22 Kelly again *displays* understanding and agrees with Sam that this is the better chart, according to her, because it is smaller than the one on her desk. However, again she perseverates: a little over four minutes later, Kelly, while walking with

---

1. Examples 1–4b, due to the nature of the setting, come from audio recordings, which means that analysis is limited to audible resources, primarily the talk. Nevertheless, revealing insights can stem from an examination of such material. Excerpts 5–7, however, come from both audio- and video-recorded interactions.

```
4.1 Reasoning with Kelly 1
Kelly Audio, 2/26/07.A, 6:10 – 6:52

01    SAM    are you able to teach anybody here?(. [ ) any
02    KLLY                                          [((cough))
03    SAM    you know have any um (0.3) students (.) to teach piano
04           to?
05    KLLY   so far nobody.
06           (0.3)
07    SAM    che[ck your- check your bag instead of that (.)
08    KLLY   [(          )
09    SAM    'cause I think they say the same thing.
10           (1.3)
11    KLLY   's (one)?
12           (5.6)
13    KLLY   Oh yeah, it does say the same thing.
14           (0.3)
15    KLLY   You're right it does.
16           (3.1)
17    KLLY   Yeah.
18           (2.1)
19    KLLY   same thing itn' it.
20    SAM    °yeah.
21           (0.3)
22    SAM    so that way (0.4)
23           because it's in there (.)
24           [you don't have to bother with getting up
25    KLLY   [(        )=
26    SAM    and checking it th[ere.
27    KLLY                     [=keep walking o[ver.
28    SAM                                      [yeah.
29           (0.4)
30    SAM    yeah.
31    KLLY   'ts true.
```

Sam around the facility starts to walk back towards her room. The conversation shown in Example 4.3 ensues.

Although Kelly continues to perseverate on the same action, Sam continues to try to reason with her to manage this "inappropriate" behavior. Similarly, a caregiver of an FTD patient is quoted by the San Francisco Gate as explaining that family members are "still trying to reason with him, but there's no reasoning with him" (Nichols, 25 February, 2007). The UCSF Memory and Aging Center's website provides practical tips for managing FTD behaviors, noting that reasoning and explanation are often futile:

> arguing or explaining is likely to make the symptoms worse, or at best, they
> won't remember or care that you argued. People with FTD often lack
> insight that their behaviors are different and problematic. Arguing with
> them logically typically does not work. Try to divert the person rather

```
4.2 Reasoning with Kelly 2
Kelly Audio, 2/26/07.A, 9:05 — 10:20

01    SAM    I have a sister.
02           (0.4)
03    KLLY   you get along with her (well)?
04           (.)
05    SAM    yea, (.) I do. very much so. >I saw< her this weekend.
06           (0.3)
07    SAM    >check-< check your bag, not- not this one
08    KLLY   check my bag?=
09    SAM    =yeah. 'cause remember it's in there?
10           (3.6)
11    KLLY   oh this one?
12    SAM    yeah.
13           (1.1)
14    KLLY   oh yeah. It's there too.
15    SAM    yeah.
16    KLLY   now I see I've g[ot (            )
17    SAM                   [ehh it's the better one.
18           (0.6)
19    KLLY   ((clear throat)) it'smaller.
20    SAM    yeah. (     ) go back once you've used that one.
21           (1.3)
22    KLLY   it's got exactly the same information on it.
23           (1.4)
24    SAM    I saw you lookin' at it during, (.) church.
25    KLLY   yeah.
```

than force him to stop a behavior. Try to redirect problem behaviors rather than force the person to stop. If a behavior is just odd but not dangerous, consider letting the person continue" (from http://memory.ucsf.edu/ftd/livingwithftd/practicaltips).

This inclination to reason with patients is quite powerful, but often unsuccessful.

Interestingly, in these examples with Kelly, the perseverative behavior itself is not treated as inappropriate; Sam does not try to reason with Kelly about why she does not need to constantly check her medication chart, but rather he tries to explain to her why a particular method of checking her medication is more appropriate or preferred than the method on which she seems reliant. He seems to understand that getting Kelly to stop perseverating is unlikely. However, there seems to be hope of diverting Kelly or getting her to perseverate on a different behavior, one which would produce the same result as her current perseverative behavior but be less disruptive in social settings; that is, when trying to maintain a conversation with her, she may feel less inclined to leave in the middle to run off to her room when an impulse strikes. Kelly, although clearly able to display understanding of the benefits of using the

```
4.3 Reasoning with Kelly 3
Kelly Audio, 2/26/07.A, 14:45 — 16:08

((Prior to this Example, Sam and Kelly are walking around the
facility in a state of incipient talk; line 1 thus begins a new
sequence))
01   SAM    whatchya doing.
02   KLLY   see if I took my heart medication.
03   SAM    oh:
04          (0.2)
05   SAM    but you have that um thing in your bag ( ) that can
06          tell you
07          (0.9)
08   KLLY   y' my chart's in there.
09   SAM    no there's the small yellow chart (0.3) remember?
10          (2.2)
11   SAM    I'll show you. when we get there.
12          (13.5) ((walking back to Kelly's room))
13   KLLY   oh, kay it is there.
14   SAM    yeah, it's (ther-) >but< also take a look inside your
15          bag.
16          (0.6)
17   SAM    'cause you'll find this yellow thing,
18          (7.4)
19   KLLY   that one?
20   SAM    yeah. and that has the same informa[tion on it
21   KLLY                                      [oh it's got the
22          same thing yeah.
23   SAM    yeah
24          (0.4)
25   SAM    so you don't have to go back here. (.) to check
26   KLLY   it's got exactly the same thi- oh [that's good. Okay,
27   SAM                                       [yeah.
28   KLLY   that's nice.
29   SAM    that way you can spend more time with the patients.
30          >Err wi' thuh: um: other res[idents.
31   KLLY                               [yeah. That's good.
32          (0.8)
33   KLLY   yeah, they say exactly the same thing.
34          (1.1)
35   KLLY   yeah so that's (a good idea to) keep it there.
36          (0.4)
```

pocket chart, is unable to appropriately shift activities when requested to do so. That she displays cognitive awareness of the benefits of Sam's alternative without behaviorally demonstrating her expressed understanding is consonant with the reports declaring that FTD patients' ability to reason and to access declarative knowledge of the social rules is still very much intact, while their ability to implement such rules is impaired. Such reasoning on the part of the caregivers, therefore, seems rather fruitless in the long-term and does not typically produce a change in behavior. In sum, there are two features of interest when observing Kelly's perseverative behaviors and how her interlocutors attempt to manage them. First, Kelly's interlocutors often attempt to reason with Kelly despite the little effect it has on her change in behavior. These reasoning practices often become more and more elaborate within the same sequence. Second, Kelly consistently displays understanding in the talk and aligns with the interlocutor's assessment of the situation, yet such understandings and alignments are rarely manifested in action.

Another point of interest is that Kelly's caregivers tried to encourage her to alter but not eliminate her perseverative behavior, a management strategy that Lough and Garfoot (2007, 304) have found to have some success. They report a case study of Mr MW who, like Kelly, showed obsessive checking behavior. His most disruptive behavior was checking the suspension of cars. He did this by rocking the car which often set off the car alarm. The authors claim that "the key to minimising the disruption caused lay in accepting that Mr MW was going to check and change the nature of the checking. This consisted of modelling a different routine using visual checking rather than rocking." They also note that "after only a few modeling sessions the checking ritual altered." In the examples above, Kelly does not alter her checking behavior even after her environment has been restructured (she is given the pocket chart to carry with her) and a more appropriate behavior was modeled for her. Questions thus arise: Do patients with different behavioral profiles respond with different success rates to modeling? Do some checking behaviors lend themselves easier to this behavioral management strategy than others? Would Kelly have been successful at altering her behavior if more systematic and more frequent modeling sessions had been conducted?

### Distraction: A quick fix

In contrast to the examples above, Example 4.4a below, although initially appearing to be similar to the others, is somewhat different. Early in this example, Sam tries again to reason with Kelly about another of her recent perseverative behaviors: using the phone. In line 37 Kelly declares that she needs to use the phone and, similar to the excerpts above, Sam tries to explain to her why she cannot. When Kelly insists, Sam reminds her that she already tried unsuccessfully to use the phone. In some ways, this explanation is an upgrade in which Sam moves from explaining a malfunction of the phone to a new line of reasoning, one that points out Kelly's past behavior to render her current request illogical. When Kelly in line 46 denies that she already tried to use the phone, Sam softly replies to the contrary (line 48); this is uttered almost as an aside, as if knowing that reasoning with her is not going to shift Kelly to a different, more socially acceptable activity. After a pause, Sam tries a new tactic to prevent her from going back to the phone. With no easy

4.4a Sam Distracting Kelly (continues from Example 3)
Kelly Audio, 2/26/07.A

```
33   KLLY    yeah, they say exactly the same thing.
34           (1.1)
35   KLLY    yeah so that's (a good idea to) keep it there.
36           (0.4)
37   KLLY    I need to go use the phone.
38           (1.6)
39    SAM    the thing is you can't because
40           'cause they only have one that k- that accepts
41           incoming calls.
42   KLLY    well, let me go check.
43           (0.5)
44    SAM    you just did though.
45           (0.6)
46   KLLY    no I didn't.
47           (1.4)
48    SAM    °yeah you did.
49           (5.1)
50    SAM    wuh tell me more about uh:
51        →  oh- who gave you those Valentine's day
52           (0.3)
53   KLLY    I don' know.
54           (0.5)
55    SAM    let's look.
56           (0.5)
57   KLLY    it says: (5.6) oh my husband.
58           (0.4)
59    SAM    ahhh (1.3) that's nice. it says to my pretty
60           little wife.
61   KLLY    that's what he always calls me.
62    SAM    really?
63   KLLY    yeah.
```

alternative behavior to suggest that would satisfy Kelly's inclination to use the phone, in lines 50–51, Sam stops trying to reason with Kelly, and changes topics altogether, asking about some flowers that Kelly has on her desk.

In line 50, Sam starts to ask Kelly to tell him more about something, but before he is able to produce a noun phrase to complete this turn, he produces a lengthened *uh:* to hold his turn until he notices the flowers. Sam then interrupts the progression of his talk with a change-of-state token, *oh*, indicating that his knowledge state has moved from a negative knowledge state to a positive knowledge state (Heritage 1984a); in other words, he makes use of a sudden noticing of an item in Kelly's room, and thus a new focus to distract Kelly. He asks about the Valentine's Day arrangement in her room, more specifically about who the flowers are from (line 51). Sam then is able to successfully redirect Kelly's behavior and maintain her focus on a new topic of conversation. This distraction is successful for nearly 40 seconds of talk in which Sam and Kelly discuss varied topics including her husband's nickname for her, dried flowers, and colorings in the room. What might make this tactic more successful than others, even if temporarily, is that Sam provides Kelly with a new focus, rather than maintain the prior framework about using the phone and asking Kelly to negotiate within it. Within that framework Kelly can easily maintain her fixation on using the phone, making it difficult for her to shift foci. However, providing a new frame, which focuses on Kelly's environment or personal belongings, allows her to orient more successfully to the shift.

In line 64 in Example 4.4b below, however, Sam starts a new sequence in which he asks about Kelly's plans for the day. The introduction of this new topic provides a context that makes relevant Kelly's response in line 65; the shift thus provides Kelly with a more appropriate context to re-engage in her perseverative activity.

Had Sam not again shifted frameworks, allowing Kelly to reinsert her desire to use the phone, who knows how long Kelly might have remained focused on these more "appropriate" topics. Interestingly, Kelly's turn in line 65 is *well*-prefaced, indicating that her response is not going to be straightforward. For example, Pomerantz (1984) and Drew (2004, 87–88) illustrate how *well* can be employed as a contrastive move in dispreferred second turns. Thus, Kelly, at some level, may recognize the problematic nature of her upcoming stated intentions or needs, yet she is either not able to or not motivated to inhibit them.

Sam is not the only interactant to employ these practices to divert Kelly's inappropriate behavior. Her husband, Bron, also uses similar practices to manage her impulses. In Example 4.5, Kelly, Bron, and a facility staff member, Rachel, are talking in Kelly's room. Kelly asks about when her piano students are scheduled for lessons (the institution where Kelly is staying is several towns from her home, so she is no longer teaching). This topic is sensitive for two reasons: 1) it is unlikely that Kelly will be able to continue teaching, and she may not be able to even return home, something Kelly is unaware of at this time, and 2) when Kelly was living at home, she continually asked about the time of her students' appointments and constantly

```
4.4b Conditional Relevance Allowing for Perseveration
Kelly Audio, 2/26/07.A (continues from Example 4a)

61   KLLY    that's what he always calls me.
62   SAM     really?
63   KLLY    yeah.
             ((30 seconds omitted))
64   SAM     mmkay, well what are your plans for today.
65   KLLY    well I need to go use the phone.
```

checked her appointment book. When Kelly first asks about her students in line 5, Bron *explains* the situation and attempts to ease her concern. When Kelly requests elaboration in lines 9–10, displaying continued concern, Bron replies with a minimal *yeah* and then immediately switches topics by asking Kelly if she missed him (this sudden topic shift in an attempt to distract Kelly seems reminiscent of parent-child interactions, see also Joaquin, Chapter 7, this volume). This pattern of management practices—moving from explanation/reasoning to a shift in topics as a distraction from the current project—is seen both in Sam and Bron's interactions with Kelly. It is interesting to notice, however, that Bron moves through this sequence of practices more quickly than did Sam, who was a less frequent interactant of Kelly's.

Similar to Example 4.4a above, this immediate distraction is fairly successful in refocusing Kelly. The interaction continues and other interactants assist in maintaining Kelly's focus on topics other than her students. Having more interactants present may allow for smoother transitions in topics. This suggests a shared sense of responsibility for the interactants to maintain a more socially appropriate conversation, one that is more or less uninterrupted by Kelly's perseverative behaviors. It is interesting to note that in all of the distractions presented by the interactants, they refocus the topic of conversation on Kelly, sometimes almost in interview-like fashion; that is, they do not attempt

```
    4.5 Bron Distracting Kelly
    Kelly 2/26/07

    01   KLLY    are we going home today or are we (staying here).
    02   BRON    well, let's find out what Becca will say you know ts
    03           jus'
    04   RACH    yeah or ( [  )
    05   KLLY              [ when are the students scheduled.
    06   BRON    (0.4) ohh, they have been (rescheduled) and once you
    07           come back we will call them an' then everything will be
    08           alright.=you don' have to worry about it at all.=
    09   KLLY    =so you jus' cancelled an' told 'em I'd call 'em when
    10           I get back?
    11   BRON    yeah.=Did you miss me?
    12   KLLY    yeah, I missed you a lot.
    13   BRON    that's nice.
    14   KLLY    Ve:ry very much.
    15   RACH    You gotta clock today.
    16           (0.5)
    17   RACH    (   ) remembered it.
    18           (2.0)
    19   RACH    where was that in your house?
    20   KLLY    this clock?
    21   RACH    yeah.
    22   KLLY    I'm not sure.
    23   RACH    was that an award that you got?
    24           (4.1) ((Kelly looking at clock))
```

to refocus her attention on someone or something that is not in some way related to her directly. This could be so for possibly two reasons: 1) Kelly is the focus of everyone's attention since she has just recently been moved to the facility and everyone came to visit her and/or 2) managing Kelly's interruptions is more successful when she is directly addressed. While these possibilities do not need to be teased apart, and indeed they both may contribute to the interactants' practices, it is important that Smith (2004, 9) also noticed in his data of two FTD patients that they were more successful at participating when the topic of conversation was directed at their immediate selves or identity. Smith states that when the topic is relevant to the patient, "the inter-subjective Gap is less difficult for the patient to bridge and necessitates less inter-subjective Work for the patient in the interaction." This also allows interactants to better manage Kelly's distracting behavior by more successfully directing her to different activities/topics unrelated to her perseverative tendencies.

### *Physically guiding the body to manage FTD behavior*

Kelly's interactants do not only use reasoning and distraction to manage Kelly's perseverative behaviors, they also physically guide her to interrupt her perseverative behaviors, particularly when the interactional goals are not centered on Kelly but on accomplishing a collaborative task involving several participants. Example 4.6 is the same interactional episode that Torrisi analyzes in this volume (presented as Example 2.3 in Chapter 2) to illustrate Kelly's "uncooperative" behavior. Here, the extract is analyzed for a different feature. (Although a different analytical focus, the two analyses in no way contradict each other.) To remind the reader of the context, I will briefly describe the setting. Kelly, along with her husband, Bron; the ethnographer, Sam; the staff member, Rachel, introduced in Example 4.5 above; another staff member, Gina; and the facility's owner and head nurse, Elinor, are present at a meeting at the facility. They are seated around a circular table. A few minutes into the meeting, Gina brings in five glasses of water on a tray, which she accidentally spills onto the table. At this point the topic of discussion comes to a halt, and everyone is now oriented to the spilled water and collaboratively attending to the activity of cleaning up and consoling Gina. Elinor, Rachel and Sam help Gina soak up the spilled water and in lines 40–41, 45 Sam tells a story of when he spilled beer in a perhaps more vulnerable setting, which is likely an attempt to make Gina feel better and take the focus off of the immediate situation. Although Kelly responds to the initial startle of the dropped glasses, she never orients to the new framework on which the others are now focused.

In this example, the public environment has been transformed. Although the transformation was not intentionally initiated by any of the interlocutors,

```
4.6 Physically Guiding Kelly
Kelly 2/26/07 00:55:25

06    SAM    it's okay. ((beginning to soak up spilled water))
07           (1.1)
08    GINA   ooo[:hh
09    ELIN       [it's jus' water. ((reaches over to pick up
10           glasses))
11           (      ) ((attending to mess))
12    RACH   he he he he he heh
13    GINA        [oh
14    SAM    it's [okay. (0.5) I've done that.
15    ELIN        [it's no problem.
16           (0.5) ((Gina turns around to get something))
17    SAM    I was a waiter. ((Kelly looking at her cookie))
18    GINA   sorry. ((whispers as she bumps camera))
19    RACH   Wake up.
20    GINA   he he I'm n(h)ot a w(hh)ai[(h)t(h)er.
21    KLLY                            [((leans to talk to Bron))
22    BRON   What?
23           (0.5)
24    GINA   (that's alright. I'll do [it.)
25    RACH                            [that's fine. ((Kelly looks at
26           Bron and her food))
27    GINA   ohhh
28    ELIN   this is why it's good you're going into nursing.
29           ((Bron points toward the others to orient Kelly))
30    BRON   ha h[a ha:
31    SAM        [>he he he he<
32    GINA   he he (.) he he
             6 seconds omitted
36    GINA   I'm fi:ne.
37           (   )
38    ELIN   (Ok, it's just) water.
39           ((Kelly stands, watching activity and still eating))
40    SAM    I've done it with lots of be:er in front of a bunch of
41           gu:[ys
42    BRON   [(sit down) sit down because it's wet (t's wet)
43           ((grabs Kelly's purse))
44    KLLY   how long are we supposed to stay here ((to Bron))
45    SAM    'n they all like cla:pped, ((gestures clapping hands))
46           'n then I was [like he he he
47                         [((Kelly sits back down))
```

it nevertheless requires those present to adjust to the new environment. Everyone successfully makes the necessary adjustments except Kelly; all the other participants reorient their bodies, moving closer to the table to ameliorate the spill and create a new framework that grounds the current shift in talk and makes new responses and actions relevant. The only attention Kelly pays to the new event is when she looks towards the fallen glasses just after the loud shattering sound (startle response). Otherwise, she pays little attention to the new activity, shifting her gaze often between her husband and the snack she is eating. This detachment from context is perhaps one of the most troublesome aspects of interacting with her; she has a great deal of difficulty adjusting to shifts in the interaction, whether it be shifts in talk or shifts in the activity or participation that are not centered on her. In line 39, Kelly stands up in an attempt to leave the table, presumably to go back to her room and check her medication chart. Given that the focus of this new framework involves a collaborative task, participants are not in a position to reason with or distract Kelly from her perseverations, in part because Kelly is not the center of this participant framework. As such, Bron employs a third management practice —physical guidance (in line 43)—which does not pull the other members' attention away from the collaborative task being oriented to. Bron, while quietly directing Kelly (line 42), grabs the strap of her purse and gently pulls until Kelly sits back down. The management practices deployed by the interlocutors are then, in part, a consequence of the larger environmental and interactional context that has emerged.

## Maintaining and Shifting Frameworks

Although commonplace, it is quite amazing how easily capable participants are of moving seamlessly in and out of changing participant frameworks (Goffman 1981, 137) given the amount of work required to do so (see C. Goodwin 1981, 2002; M. Goodwin 1997). As these frameworks emerge and dissolve, participants take up new roles, adjust their talk, and reorient their physical bodies to adapt to the changing interactive demands, which can be slight or, as in Example 4.6, more radical. The crash of glasses alone is enough to beckon an additional staff member from a different location to the room who then assists with this new activity of cleaning up. Although shifting activities and participant frameworks is difficult for Kelly, she does seem capable of shifting more comfortably within changing physical environments. In one afternoon I accompanied her to the hospital for an fMRI, to her hotel, to a restaurant for dinner, and back to the hotel, all in a city relatively unfamiliar to her. She had no apparent difficulties with the drastically different physical structures and environments. Rather her trouble came only during the more local interactions within these environments. For instance, in the restaurant, she seemed to possess a general schema; she knew to look at the menu to find a selection, she knew to order and to place her order with the server. However, she showed difficulty telling the server what she wanted in a socially expected and thus acceptable way. The server attempted to take drink orders first but Kelly continued to tell the server her meal order even while she was taking drink orders from the others. When the meal orders did become relevant, Kelly repeats hers several times.

In Example 4.6, Kelly does not successfully re-orient to the new participant framework or collaborative activity. The body displays of the interactants make it clear to what they are now attending: the spilled glasses of water. One of the ramifications of this is that, if true, it seems that the very behaviors that affect individuals with FTD also cause them to be removed from the general public. Their actions publicly display mental states, which allow for others to first infer from those states an evident course of action and thereby coordinate action with multiple (in this case six) participants and accomplish a larger goal. Kelly, however, never attends to the new activity: she never gazes with interest toward the focused task, never attempts to help or participate. Rather in line 39, she disengages by standing up and moving away from the table. Bron's physical guidance of Kelly in line 43 places her in a more socially expected position, that is, a position closer to the activity on which everyone is focused. Although Kelly never becomes a participating member, Bron is able to at least maintain her presence at the table, which places her in a position to more easily "blend in" to the collaborative activity being negotiated. C. Goodwin (2002, 39) remarks that, even when disengaged from a local spate of talk, participants can maintain mutual orientation to the "encounter as a whole" by positioning the lower portion of their body towards their participant (this was discussed in a two-person activity). In Example 4.6, Kelly disengages both from the local talk with her eye gaze and head position and from the larger encounter with her redirected lower body and movement away from the table. Bron, perhaps knowing that asking Kelly to engage appropriately in the task will be ineffective, tries to put Kelly in a physical position where she could be seen as showing engagement to the encounter as a whole. She therefore needs assistance to, at the very least, remain superficially involved.

Kelly is not the only patient diagnosed with FTD who demonstrates difficulty maintaining and shifting frameworks to which caregivers' respond with physical guidance. Another patient, Romeo, a 63-year old male, diagnosed approximately two years earlier also demonstrates perseverative behaviors: he repeatedly requests the TV to be turned on and off and walks from the living room to the kitchen repeatedly to reheat coffee. Because these behaviors typically occur at home and in private, they cause less interference in social situations and therefore require less management on the part of his wife and primary caregiver, Juliet. However, when in public settings, Juliet, does manage Romeo's behavior so that he is participating in socially expected ways. In Example 4.7, Romeo and Juliet are in the drugstore. Juliet and Romeo approach the pharmacy line, which is delimited by two ropes supported by four poles. Juliet walks between the ropes and Romeo follows her. She then moves to sit down in a chair next to the line while uttering line 1 (Juliet has just had back surgery).

In Example 4.7, Romeo seems to have trouble shifting to a new activity. Juliet, in lines 6–7, must not only orient him to the new activity of waiting in line, but must also assist him in what he will need for the future shift in tasks. What is striking about Romeo is that, unlike Kelly, he displays his apparent awareness of his difficulty making these shifts smoothly. For instance, in line 4 he indicates that he is not certain to what activity he is to attend. That is, Romeo seems to be aware that waiting is not the activity to which he will be attending in the future, but it is unclear to him what the future activity will require; in this case, he seems aware that a credit card is one required item relevant to this context (line 9). Similar to Kelly's understanding of the overall purpose of the restaurant, Romeo seems to have a general schema for stores, but shifting smoothly between tasks in order to carry out the schema is problematic. Once the line waiting activity has been established and Romeo can orient to it, he successfully waits for over two minutes. However, when the cashier in line 18 provides the next move to shift frameworks—*Sir, I can help you down here*—Romeo does not engage in the larger interactive field of this sub-activity but rather remains focused on the immediate task of waiting in line. When the man waiting behind Romeo

```
4.7 Physically Guiding Romeo, Line Waiting
Romeo 1/17/07


01    JLT    Can you stand there? I'm gonna sit for a moment.
02    JLT    ((Juliet sighs as she sits down in chair))
03           (0.9)
04    ROM    ((turns to look at Juliet)) now what.
05           (2.1)
06    JLT    just wait our turn. ((Romeo returns to face front))
07           we're waiting our turn.
08           (3.2)
09    ROM    (you wan' me to) use the credit card?
10           (0.5)
11    JLT    yeah.
12           ((Romeo opens wallet))
13    JLT    >ya don' need to bring it out yet<, Romeo.
14           ((Romeo still attending to wallet))
15    JLT    Romeo, ya don' need to bring it out yet.
16           (0.6)
17    ROM    kay. ((closes wallet))
             2 minutes 20 seconds of line waiting
18    EMPL   Sir, I can help you down here.
19    JLT    that's us. ((man behind Romeo start to move around to
20           go to cashier))
21        →  ((grabbing Romeo's jacket and directs him forward))
22           We're next. We-we: were next.
23              [Sorry.
24    MAN    go [ahead. I'm (       ) no problem.
```

starts to move around him, Juliet acts to claim their place in line. In doing so, she interrupts Romeo's fixed orientation to the current task of line waiting. She does this by publicly announcing to the other customers who are waiting in line that they were next, and she grabs Romeo's jacket to physically guide him toward the pharmacist's window. Similar to the way Bron physically guided Kelly to keep her oriented to the current framework, Juliet physically directs Romeo so he appears to be attending to the new task to which the line waiting served as a sub-goal. While Romeo's behaviors in this interaction are not perseverative as Kelly's had been in the previous extracts, they do demonstrate mental rigidity that prevents him from shifting tasks smoothly just as Kelly's perseverative behaviors keep her from seamlessly shifting tasks or maintaining focus on current tasks.

## The Benefits of Examining Naturally Occurring FTD Interactions and Reflections on Caregiver Stress

Most studies of FTD and frontal lobe dysfunction examine perseverative behaviors including perseverative errors on various tasks in controlled, experimental settings. These studies rarely describe perseveration as it relates specifically to the reported social incompetence of FTD. Some studies aim to find if perseveration is a diagnostic feature that can distinguish FTD from other dementias such as Alzheimer's disease, while others focus on the neurobiological underpinnings of such behavior. For instance, perseveration has been found to be more strongly associated with right frontal lobe functioning than with left frontal lobe functioning (Boone *et al.* 1999, 620). These studies are important and necessary; however, ethnomethodological approaches to FTD can also illuminate aspects of FTD behavior, particularly those aspects that relate to caregiver concerns. Some caregivers have even reported their frustration with the lack of more extensive and systematic observation. One caregiver, for instance, told a reporter, "I wish these people [experts] had more time to observe. I'm not sure they're getting a full picture" (Nichols, 25 February, 2007). Direct observation through ethnographic methods and CA can help construct a fuller picture. The next section discusses the potential benefits of this approach as it relates specifically to the data examined in this chapter.

### Perseverative Behaviors in Real-time and in the Real World

"Numerous factors mediate carer burden, including the severity of the cognitive impairment, the degree of behavioural disturbance and the difficulties of undertaking specific caregiving tasks" (Lough and Garfoot 2007, 286). Embarrassment associated with commonly reported gross inappropriate behaviors such as inappropriate touching are certainly a source of stress and anxiety for caregivers and other family members. The behavioral profile of FTD is different from other dementias that do not usually present with the severity of psychiatric and behavioral symptoms and antisocial behaviors (Lough and Garfoot 2007, 301). Perseverative behaviors, like those exhibited by Kelly, also surely take a toll on caregivers. These and similar behaviors may place the greatest strain or burden on caregivers because they are exhibited so frequently. The frequency at which perseverative behaviors can take place was illustrated above in Examples 4.1-4.4b. Following Example 4.1, for instance, only two minutes and 23 seconds elapsed before Kelly again attempted to check her medication chart. Her perseverative behavior continually disrupted the flow of the interaction, which caregivers often attempt to retain, a responsibility which likely leads to caregiver stress. Caregiver stress is probably caused not only because of the frequency of such behaviors, but also because of their overall effect on the current interaction.

As we saw above, Kelly's perseverative behaviors can and typically do dominate the interaction. For instance, her initiations of a perseverative behavior often launch a lengthy sequence in which participants attempt to either reason with Kelly, provide her an alternative behavior, and/or divert her attention away from the perseverative behavior. The work required by her interlocutors to accomplish these aims, regardless of whether or not they are successful, is evident in the extracts above. In the first four extracts alone, which were drawn from only 25 minutes of recorded interaction, Kelly's interlocutors spend approximately three minutes addressing her perseverations. While this may not appear to be a long time, these three minutes were not consecutive. Thus, as was mentioned above, the conversation that was in progress repeatedly came to a halt and thus, on many occasions throughout the conversation, required everyone else to suspend his/her interactional goals. That very few interactants could successfully complete their own interactional goals is consonant with the description of FTD patients as being self-centered and uncaring (Mendez 2006, 412), which Lough and Garfoot (2007, 302) note is often the case because when reasoning is unsuccessful, interactants perceive patients' behavior to be intentional. Perseverative behaviors are quite certainly frustrating to interactants, especially to primary caregivers who likely feel the most responsibility to control them and keep interactions progressing in a more expected and collaborative manner.

### Caregiver Management Practices

Another source of caregiver stress regarding perseverative behaviors may be due to the fact that there is not a simple or clear successful strategy for managing them like there are for other kinds of behaviors. During interviews conducted by our research team, caregivers often reported conscious strategies that they use to manage inappropriate behaviors. These strategies tended to be quite concrete and often centered on safety, for example, hiding knives, locking doors, and prohibiting the use of the oven. However, caregivers were less likely to be conscious of or able to articulate management practices they employed in natural interaction, especially discourse practices. This distinction between types of practices (i.e., practices addressing dangerous behaviors and those addressing interactional norms) is reminiscent of Sacks' description of the two kinds of rules adults give to children: class 1 rules for which the consequences result naturally from the act (e.g., getting burned after touching a stove) and class 2 rules which require an observer for negative consequences to be endured (e.g., lying and perhaps perseverative behaviors) (Sacks 1992, vol 1, 78–79). This parallel is interesting because FTD patients are often described as childlike (see Joaquin, Chapter 7, this volume for other parallels between the behavior of FTD patients and children) and also because class 1 rules seem to be considerably easier for patients to follow than class 2 rules, revealing patients' difficulty with socially embedded constraints. Additionally, while caregivers often report the prevalence and topical focus of compulsive or perseverative behaviors, they rarely recount whether they employ recurring practices to manage such behaviors or the degree of their effectiveness. The use of CA, in part because it insists on audio and/or video recording, allows one to inspect carefully and repeatedly the ways in which caregivers organically respond to perseverative behaviors (or some other deviance) and to follow moment-by-moment how patients react to such responses. With this methodology, one can determine whether or not caregiver practices are able to deter, inhibit, or prevent the behavior they are addressing.

Whether or not caregivers are aware of the impact of their management practices, they use them even when they have seemingly little effect. Caregivers reveal a need to address the perseverative behavior in some way. These attempts, which frequently end in failure and likely frustration, show that caregivers are highly concerned about maintaining the integrity of an interaction and are likely under much stress to try to do so. Further burden stems from the loss of sense of control a caregiver inevitably confronts in such situations (Lough and Garfoot 2007, 302). Additionally, caregivers' persistence shows the power of conditional relevance, which is summarized by Sacks *et al.* (1974, 728) who state, "generally, a turn's talk will be heard as directed to a prior turn's talk, unless special techniques are used to locate some other talk to which it is directed" (see below for further discussion). Interlocutors are so oriented to understanding and demonstrating the conditional relevance of another's turn, that even when the turn is disruptive to the ongoing progressivity of the current course of action, as is the case in many interactions with FTD patients, caregivers make an effort to address the patient's turn or integrate it into the course of the current talk.

## The Interaction Order: Caregivers' Attempts to Preserve Conditional Relevance

Examining how interlocutors manage perseverative behaviors of and initiate appropriate behavior from FTD patients illuminates interactional features that interlocutors find important to preserve in the structure or social order of interaction, what Goffman called "the interaction order" (Goffman 1983). Interlocutors' attempts to reason with Kelly to stop her perseverative behaviors show how they initially treat Kelly as a fully (i.e., addressed) ratified participant, that is, "oriented to by the speaker in a manner to suggest that his words are particularly for them, and that some answer is therefore anticipated from them" (Goffman 1981, 9–10). They frequently treat her turns as deserving of a conditionally relevant and paired response [i.e., a matched second pair part (SPP) to Kelly's first pair part (FPP) (see Schegloff and Sacks 1973, 295–296 for a description of the adjacency pair apparatus including pair parts)]. Responding in a way that is conditionally relevant to Kelly's perseverative turns at talk, not only demonstrates the powerful expectations of producing turns that are responsive and designed for one's recipient (Sacks *et al.* 1974), it also reveals the importance of maintaining topics, which often transition in a step-wise fashion (Jefferson 1984) or are marked at turn beginnings if abrupt (e.g., with *oh* to show that the turn came to the speaker suddenly or *by the way* to demonstrate that the turn may be out of place). Of course, the only way to produce a conditionally relevant SPP to one of Kelly's FPPs and to progress the current topic put forth by Kelly is to treat her as a fully functioning and ratified member of the conversation and to treat her turns at talk as relevant. The fact that Kelly displays an understanding and ability to reason with her interlocutors likely makes it easier for her interlocutors to, at least initially, uphold the expectations of conditional relevance and topic maintenance.

The power of maintaining conditional relevance is evident even when interlocutors attempt a new discourse practice to distract Kelly and refocus her attention on something unrelated to her perseverative tendencies. For instance, in Examples 4.4a and 4.5 (portions of which are reproduced below as Examples 4.8 and 4.9), Sam and Bron still close the sequence that is dealing with Kelly's concerns about making a phone call (in Example 4.8) or scheduling students (in Example 4.9) before shifting topics.

In line 12 of Example 4.8, Sam treats Kelly's prior turn (*no I didn't*) as deserving of a conditionally relevant response even though his next move indicates that he knows this line of reasoning is likely to be unproductive. He

```
4.8 Sam Maintaining Conditional Relevance
Kelly 2/26/07 (portion of Example 4a)


03   SAM    the thing is you can't because
04          'cause they only have one that k- that accepts
05          incoming calls.
06   KLLY   well, let me go check.
07          (0.5)
08   SAM    you just did though.
09          (0.6)
10   KLLY   no I didn't.
11          (1.4)
12   SAM    °yeah you did.
13          (5.1)
14   SAM    wuh tell me more about uh:
15          oh- who gave you those Valentine's day
16          (0.3)
17   KLLY   I don' know.
```

does not suddenly abandon the sequence in progress to try to distract Kelly from her perseverative goals. Rather after a 5.1 second silence,[2] he attempts to distract her by beginning a new sequence.

Although Bron moves much more quickly from the reasoning to distraction practice in Example 4.9, he still responds to Kelly's FPP before attempting to distract Kelly. Kelly asks a yes-no question in lines 9–10 which makes conditionally relevant a *yes* or *no* response and requires Bron to confirm information he has already given. Bron does not ignore Kelly's question or treat it explicitly as inappropriate, but instead provides the conditionally relevant response (a no problem response) before quickly producing a new FPP to distract Kelly and prevent her from extending the prior sequence. The practices of Kelly's interlocutors demonstrate the strong expectations of conditional relevance in natural conversation. Regardless of how they attempt to manage her perseverative tendencies (whether by reasoning/explanation or by distraction), they rarely disregard the expectation of conditional relevance.

Kelly's perseverative behaviors, on the other hand, often disregard the expectations of conditional relevance. For instance, Sam and Kelly made plans to take a walk around the facility and as they were walking, Kelly starts to turn back, thereby disregarding the plans that had just been made with Sam. In conversation, Kelly also disregards such expectations. For example, in Example 4.5 (part of which is reproduced opposite as Example 4.10), Kelly introduces a new FPP in line 5 that interrupts Rachel's turn in progress (in line 4) and abandons the sequence.

---

2.   Because this extract was only audio-recorded, it is not clear what is happening actionally during this silence.

```
4.9 Bron Maintaining Conditional Relevance
Kelly 2/26/07 (portion of Example 5)

05  KLLY                 [ when are the students scheduled.
06  BRON    (0.4) ohh, they have been (rescheduled) and once you
07          come back we will call them an' then everything will be
08          alright.=you don' have to worry about it at all.=
09  KLLY    =so you jus' cancelled an' told 'em I'd call 'em when
10          I get back?
11  BRON→   yeah.=Did you miss me?
12  KLLY    yeah, I missed you a lot.
13  BRON    that's nice.
```

Kelly's response is neither directed to Rachel's turn nor does it employ any special device to show how it is directed to some other turn. While Kelly's perseverative behaviors are unresponsive to others' turns and interactional aims, caregivers often exert quite a bit of effort to be responsive to Kelly's turns to maintain the current interactional framework.

## Conclusion: Disruptions of Progressivity and Displays of Understanding in FTD Interactions

Whether best described as perseverance, difficulty in shifting sets, and/ or mental rigidity, what seems to be common to both Kelly and Romeo's examined behaviors is their effects on the *progressivity* of the current course of action. Kelly and Romeo's behaviors often interrupt the progression of the sequence. Kelly's perseverative tendencies often prompt participants to redirect their interactive goals to the task of stopping her perseverative behaviors, which requires them to put their own interactive goals on hold or abandon them altogether. Romeo initiates very few spontaneous behaviors, and participants often respond to him by attempting to prompt him to participate in the current goals of the interactants. Whether caregivers attempted to stop inappropriate behaviors or initiate appropriate behaviors, such disruptions of the progressivity of activity were treated as in need of 'fixing.'

From the examination of Kelly's perseverative behaviors, one finds that she

```
4.10 Kelly Disregarding Conditional Relevance
Kelly 2/26/07 (portion of Example 5)

01  KLLY    are we going home today or are we (staying here).
02  BRON    well, let's find out what Becca will say you know ts
03          jus'
04  RACH    yeah or ( [  )
05  KLLY                 [ when are the students scheduled.
06  BRON    (0.4) ohh, they have been (rescheduled) and once you
07          come back we will call them an' then everything will be
08          alright.=you don' have to worry about it at all.=
```

often produces appropriate discourse responses to her interlocutors' attempts to reason with her. That is, she *displays* understanding of her interlocutors' reasoning, which perhaps provides them with evidence that she is also capable of *demonstrating* understanding (see also Mikesell 2008, 2009 for examples of a different patient, SD, who similarly displays understanding which he does not demonstrate when required). As briefly mentioned above, FTD patients, at least in the early stages of dementia, have good cognitive functioning and intact reasoning skills. They are able to reason about social rules even though they have difficulty putting these rules into action. This dissociation is seen in Kelly's ability to display understanding or awareness of another's reasoning and her tendency to not demonstrate this understanding in action.

A consequence of this is that in interactions that are brief or structured, participants might see a cooperative side of the patient where the interactional context requires only a *display* in understanding. In institutional settings like the clinical interview, for example, patients may be asked series of questions to which they must respond briefly, and they usually show their knowledge about their history or life situation. For example, when one patient in our study, Steve, was first taken to see a doctor, the doctor concluded from her interview that nothing seemed to be wrong, specifically noting that Steve was able to provide details about his life. In clinical contexts, patients are less often put in situations that require them to participate in collaborative or goal-oriented activity where they are required to *use* this knowledge demonstratively. As such, their deficits are less likely to be revealed without direct observation in naturalistic settings and over a longer period of time, at least in early stages. Another implication of this finding is that displays of understanding, in the absence of their demonstration, may be an isolatable feature that helps to more precisely define the core diagnostic feature: "early impairment of regulation of personal conduct." While there are likely several isolatable features that have led to this one diagnostic criterion, understanding the aforementioned disassociation between displaying and demonstrating appropriateness may help elucidate it.

## References

Boone, K.B., B.L. Miller, A. Lee, N. Berman, D. Sherman and D.T. Stuss.

1999 Neuropsychological patterns in right versus left frontotemporal dementia. *Journal of the International Neuropsychological Society* 5: 616–622.

Drew, P.

2004 Conversation analysis. In *Handbook of language and social interaction*, edited by K.L. Fitch and R.E. Sanders, 71–102. Lawrence Erlbaum.

Goffman, E.

1981 *Forms of talk*. Philadelphia: University of Pennsylvania Press.

1983 The interaction order: American Sociological Association 1982 presidential address. *American Sociological Review* 48(1): 1–17.

Goodwin, C.

1981 *Conversational organization: Interaction between speakers and hearers*. New York: Academic Press.

2002 Time in action. *Current Anthropology* 43: S19–S35.

Goodwin, M.H.

1997 By-play: Negotiating evaluation in storytelling. In *Towards a social science of language: Papers in honor of William Labov 2: Social interaction and discourse structures*, edited by G.R. Guy, C.Feagin, D. Schiffrin and J. Baugh, 77–102. Philadelphia, PA: John Benjamins.

Harding, N. and Palfrey, C.

1997 *The social construction of dementia: Confused professionals?* London: Jessica Kingsley.

Heritage, J.

1984a A change of state token and aspects of its sequential placement. In *Structures of social action: Studies in conversation analysis*, edited by J.M. Atkinson and J. Heritage, 299–345. Cambridge: Cambridge University Press.

1984b *Garfinkel and ethnomethodology*. Cambridge: Polity Press.

Heritage, J. and Atkinson, J. M.

1984 Introduction. In *Structures of social action: Studies in conversation analysis*, edited by J. M. Atkinson and J. Heritage, 1–16. Cambridge: Cambridge University Press.

Jagust, W.J., B.R. Reed, J.P. Seab, J.H. Kramer and T.F. Budinger.

1989 Clinical-physiologic correlates of Alzheimer's disease and frontal lobe dementia. *American Journal of Physiological Imaging* 4(3): 89–96.

Jefferson, G.

1984 On step-wise transition from talk about a trouble to inappropriately next-positioned matters. In *Structures of social action*, edited by J.M. Atkinson and J. Heritage, 191–222. Cambridge: Cambridge University Press.

Lough, S. and V. Garfoot.

2007 Psychological interventions in frontotemporal dementia. In *Frontotemporal dementia syndromes*, edited by J.R. Hodges, 277–325. Cambridge: Cambridge University Press.

Maynard, D.W. and S.E. Clayman.

1991  The diversity of ethnomethodology. *Annual Review of Sociology* 17: 385–418.

Mendez, M.F.

2006  What frontotemporal dementia reveals about the neurobiological basis of morality. *Medical Hypotheses* 67: 411–418.

Mendez, M.F., A. McMurtray, K. Chen, J.S. Shapira, F. Mishkin and B.L. Miller.

2005  Functional neuroimaging and presenting psychiatric features in frontotemporal dementia. *Journal of Neurology, Neurosurgery, and Psychiatry* 77: 4–7.

Mikesell, L.

2008  Conversational practices of a frontotemporal dementia patient: Negotiating turns, getting lost in sequences. Poster presented at the Center for Culture, Language and Interaction Conference, University of Los Angeles, California.

2009  Conversational practices of a frontotemporal dementia patient and his interlocutors. *Research on Language and Social Interaction* 42(2): 1–28.

Miller, B.L., W.W. Seeley, P. Mychack, H.J. Rosen, I. Mena and K. Boone.

2001  Neuroanatomy of the self: Evidence from patients with frontotemporal dementia. *Neurology* 57: 817–821.

Molloy, W.D. and R. Lubinski.

1991  Dementia: Impact and clinical perspectives. In *Dementia and communication,* edited by R. Lubinski, 2–21. Philadelphia, PA: B. C. Decker.

Neary, D., J.S. Snowden, L. Gustafson, U. Passant, D. Stuss, S. Black, S. Freedman, A. Kertesz, , P.H. Robert, M. Albert, K. Boone, B.L. Miller, J. Cummings and D.F. Benson.

1998  Frontotemporal lobar degeneration: A consensus on clinical diagnostic criteria. *Neurology* 51(6): 1546–1554.

Nichols, K.

2007  The other dementia. *San Francisco Chronicle.* (February 25, 2007). Retrieved on 14 December 2008 from http://www.sfgate.com/cgi-bin/article.cgi?f=/c/a/2007/02/25/CMGSQNSC8F1.DTL&hw=the+other+dementia&sn=002&sc=508

Osimani, A. and M. Freedman.

1991  Functional anatomy. In *Dementia and communication,* edited by R. Lubinski, 22–36. Philadelphia: B. C. Decker.

Pomerantz, A.

1984 Agreeing and disagreeing with assessments: Some features of preferred/dispreferred turn shapes. In *Structures of social action: Studies in conversation analysis,* edited by J.M. Atkinson and J. Heritage, 57–101. Cambridge: Cambridge University Press.

Sacks, H.

1992 *Lectures on conversation,* volume 1. Edited by G. Jefferson. Oxford: Blackwell.

Sacks, H., A.E. Schegloff and G. Jefferson.

1974 A simplest systematics for the organization of turn-taking for conversation. *Language* 50: 696–735.

Schegloff, E.A. and H. Sacks.

1973 Opening up closings. *Semiotica* 7: 289–327.

Smith, M.S.

2004 Frontotemporal dementia: The ethnomethodology of a neurological disease. Unpublished honors thesis, University of California, Los Angeles.

Ulatowska, H.K. and S.B. Chapman.

1991 Discourse studies. In *Dementia and communication,* edited by R. Lubinski, 115–132. Philadelphia, PA: B.C. Decker.

University of California, San Francisco Memory and Aging Center. A Documentary Film. Retrieved 3 March 2007 from http://www.memory.ucsf.edu/Documentary_Site/film.html

University of California, San Francisco Memory and Aging Center. Living with FTD: Practical Tips. Retrieved 2 January 2009 from http://memory.ucsf.edu/ftd/livingwithftd/practicaltips

— 5 —

# The Interactive Organization of "Insight": Clinical Interviews with Frontotemporal Dementia Patients

Netta Avineri

One of the most striking features of Frontotemporal Dementia (FTD) is "early loss of insight," which is one of the five diagnostic criteria of the disease (Neary *et al.* 2005, 772). Neary *et al.* (1998, 1550) define "early loss of insight" as a "lack of awareness of mental symptoms, evidenced by frank denial of symptoms or unconcern about the social, occupational, and financial consequences of mental failure." This chapter considers how clinicians attempt to locate insight (or its loss) through question design during medical interactions and how patients do or do not demonstrate insight through their responses. Through a detailed analysis of one doctor-patient interaction, which highlights the complex interactional manifestations of insight, this chapter will consider the fact that the current clinical definition for "early loss of insight" may be an insufficient diagnostic criterion. Traditionally, "insight" has been understood as something an individual has about oneself, but in fact insight may be something that is collaboratively established by multiple parties. This analysis also illuminates issues of epistemic authority, self-awareness, and intersubjectivity in clinical interaction more generally.

## What Does "Loss of Insight" Look Like?

In order to demonstrate the concept of insight in the clinic, I will briefly introduce an excerpt that would be argued to demonstrate a lack of insight. The following example includes the doctor (DOC2), the patient (ELIZ), and the patient's husband (sitting next to ELIZ during the interaction).

```
5.1 Pick's Disease
Elizabeth Clinic Visit

01  DOC2    Can you tell me a little bit why y(er) see Dr. Jackson?
02          Why? is it that you come to visit us.
03          (1.5) ((ELIZ looks to the side and adjusts bra strap))
04  ELIZ    I have Pick's deesease. ((Grabs arms of chair with both
05          hands and moves body up and down in seat, adjusts
06          watch as DOC2 begins to talk))
07  DOC2    You have Pick's disease (0.2) °okay.° ((Nods head)) And
08          because of that what (0.2) ((moves chair back)) what
09          have you noticed. (.) from the Pick's disease.
10          (0.4)
11  ELIZ    Nothing.
12  DOC2    Nothing at all.
13          (2.0) ((ELIZ stares at DOC2))
14  DOC2    It's the same person. (0.2) No problems: no memory
15           proble:ms or anything else?
16          0.5)
17  ELIZ    Yes.
18  DOC2    Yeah. (.) Okay. How have you been feeling lately.
19          (0.2)
20  ELIZ    Fine.
21  DOC2    Good. Okay. (.) Um:. Tsk tell me a little bit about
22          what you used to do for work.
23          (2.0)
24  ELIZ    I was (sk) former school teacher.
```

In the previous excerpt, the patient acknowledges that she has Pick's disease (another term for FTD) at line 4, but does not acknowledge any problems associated with the condition (line 11). The patient's one-word responses and absence of elaboration seem insufficient, for the patient does not take a stance towards the questions or responses. Also, the doctor abandons the issue of insight fairly quickly after receiving a "No problem" response from Elizabeth. One issue to consider is whether this short exchange would provide enough evidence to conclude that she does in fact lack insight. Another question one could reflect upon is what may have happened had the clinician pursued the issue of insight with further questions. In the rest of this chapter, I will explore what happens when a physician does pursue the issue of insight and how complex its manifestations can become when this occurs.

## The Aim of this Chapter

The aim of this chapter is to consider how "loss of insight" may or may not be an observable feature of FTD in the clinic. More specifically, if one focuses on the sequential organization of and the relationships between questions and responses, as opposed to focusing exclusively on the content of the doctor's and patient's utterances, one can begin to observe the interactional manifestations of insight. This chapter will consider alternatives to the ways insight can be conceived, operationalized, and used in the clinic. In so doing, it seeks to broaden perspectives on insight, such that more of what patients *are* able to do is acknowledged, aspects that may presently be hidden due to the current modes of operating with these patients within the clinical setting. The present research serves as a complement to the extensive work being undertaken in naturally-occurring interactions in the home and other settings, as described in the other chapters in this book.

## FTD and Insight

As Rankin *et al.* (2005, 632) highlight, "Consensus guidelines for FTD emphasize early behavioural change as a feature of the disease, along with disinhibition, impulsive or inappropriate behaviour, difficulty in modulating behaviour, and other large departures from premorbid personality. In addition, patients are noted to show little insight or self awareness regarding these changes." Frequently, as Rabins *et al.* (2006, 15) point out, dementia patients' family members are the primary individuals to first observe the "forgetfulness, communication difficulty, problems in functioning…or personality change[s]" associated with the disease. In addition, in their study of unawareness in FTD and Alzheimer's Disease (AD) patients, Salmon *et al.* (2008, 176) highlight the fact that in general "caregivers assessed symptoms more severely than patients did." In some cases, the caregivers also notice that the patient does not recognize any changes or problems him/herself, which may be one reason for bringing the patient in to the doctor for the first time. During routine visits, in addition to administering tests such as the Mini-Mental State Exam (MMSE) and asking FTD patients a number of other questions, clinicians frequently ask at least a few questions related to the patient's insight.

Researchers have attempted to operationalize "insight" through a number of measures. Rankin *et al.* (2005) and Salmon *et al.* (2007) both gave FTD and AD patients questionnaires in order to measure their unawareness of symptoms related to the disease. In both studies, FTD patients were found to have less awareness of personality changes than their age-matched AD controls. In *Loss of Insight and Functional Neuroimaging in Frontotemporal Dementia*, Mendez and Shapira (2005) report the results from questionnaires ("the UCLA FTD Insight Scale") that were administered to patients in an attempt to measure the patients' insight into their disease. They found that patients given the *UCLA FTD Insight Scale* "could not convey a commensurate concern about the consequences of their behavioral symptoms and usually felt that these symptoms did not represent disturbances, abnormalities, or significant changes from their usual patterns of behavior" (Mendez and Shapira 2005, 414).

O'Keeffe *et al.* (2007, 653), in their consideration of loss of insight in frontotemporal dementia, corticobasal degeneration and progressive supranuclear palsy, used a "multidimensional approach" to measure loss of insight. This approach examined "metacognitive knowledge of the disorders, online monitoring of errors (emergent awareness) and ability to accurately predict performance on future tasks (anticipatory awareness)." All of these measures, while able to pinpoint certain aspects of this feature of the disease, are not necessarily able to identify the more subtle aspects of how insight does or does not manifest itself interactionally.

Evers *et al.* (2007, 15) investigated the usefulness of the notion of insight in FTD diagnoses. In this article, they distinguished among three levels of insight :

1. *State awareness.* Insight into one's own states, e.g., awareness of the fact that one's physical or mental condition is altered from earlier conditions. In its absence, one is unaware and possibly in a state of denial of alterations and fails to see a problem.

2. *Illness awareness.* Insight into the fact that one's condition is altered in a manner implying illness. In its absence, the patient may be aware of a problem, but does not interpret it symptomatically as a sign of illness.

3. *Medical awareness.* Insight into the fact that the altered condition is an illness caused by given factors. Since lack of medical knowledge can hardly be a criterion of illness, level three is only of interest in this context when present.

In their work with eight FTD patients, they noted that "insight was present in three out of eight patients, and that insight appears to be a heterogeneous concept. Two types of insight emerged: Emotional insight associated with frontotemporal functions, and cognitive insight, related to posterior cognitive functions" (Evers *et al.* 2007, 13). In their description of insight as a multi-faceted concept, Evers *et al.*'s distinctive work touches on many issues relevant to the present topic.

This analysis will explore the notion that in addition to the components of insight currently included in the clinical definition *and* those considered by Evers *et al.* (2007), insight also includes an understanding of the knowledge others may have about you (which you may or may not share). Though this is information that questionnaires may be able to establish on the surface, it is primarily during clinical interactions, especially those with copresent caregivers, that this aspect of insight would manifest itself. This chapter explores this aspect of insight by analyzing one patient's interaction with her treating neurologist and caregiver in the controlled setting of the medical clinic, in an effort to better understand the construction of insight and its utility as an observable feature of FTD.

## FTD and Theory of Mind

As the examples in this chapter will demonstrate, the FTD patient is able to recognize that others may have a different perspective on her condition than she does. This finding is closely related to the notion of theory of mind, "a person's ability to understand that another person has his or her own unique way of thinking and feeling" (Boyd 2008, 366). There have been a number of studies that have explored the notion of Theory of Mind (ToM) within the FTD population (Eslinger *et al.* 2007; Gregory *et al.* 2002; Kipps and Hodges 2006; Lough *et al.* 2006), based primarily on tests administered to patients to determine which categories of Theory of Mind have been affected. Kipps and Hodges (2006, 238) have established that FTD patients' performance on the majority of Theory of Mind assessments is negatively affected, as illustrated in Table 5.1 below. They also highlight the fact that "ToM is abnormal in FTD, but that some aspects of ToM processing are more disrupted than others (affective more than cognitive)" (242).

A number of researchers establish a connection between FTD patients' impaired performance on Theory of Mind measures and their social impairment and are thus investigating specific features of both Theory of Mind and social impairment in an effort to determine which are most correlated (e.g., Gregory *et al.* 2002). For example, based on research in Fernandez-Duque *et al.* (2009) in which it is demonstrated that "a conceptual deficit in theory of mind—as measured by the false-belief task—is not at the core of the differences between bvFTD and AD, Fernandez-Duque argues against theory-of-mind impairment, as measured by the false-belief task, as the major contributor to social dysfunction of FTD patients (http://www18.

| Test | Performance |
|---|---|
| First-order ToM | mildly affected |
| Second-order ToM | mildly affected |
| Faux pas | moderately affected |
|    Cognitive | moderately affected |
|    Affective | markedly affected |
| Empathy | markedly affected |
| Mind in the eyes | moderately affected |
| Social rules | not affected |
| Social violations | moderately affected |
| Moral-conventional distinctions | moderately affected |
| Mental state verbs | mildly affected |
| Emotion recognition | moderately affected |
| Disinhibition | markedly affected |
| Executive function | not affected to markedly affected |

Table 5.1    Theory of mind (ToM) and related tests in bvFTD.

homepage.villanova.edu/diego.fernandezduque/). A number of studies have also stressed the importance of developing and utilizing ecologically valid ToM tests. As Gregory *et al.* (2002, 761) note, "at present, the diagnosis of fvFTD often depends almost entirely upon relative/carer reports of change in personality and social comportment…There is clearly a need for tasks that are capable of measuring alterations in social cognition." Lough *et al.* (2006, 956) state, "future studies should attempt to more accurately replicate the real-time dynamic that is implicit in social interactions by attempting more 'ecological' methods of testing." The present analysis seeks to demonstrate that the patient is able to display elements of Theory of Mind throughout the clinical interview, elements that may not necessarily become evident through ToM tests that are currently utilized.

## Doctor-patient Interaction: The Structure of Medical Visits

As ten Have (2005, 138) notes, "medical encounters are tightly organized events" that conform to a specific mode of organization (partially) independent of the details of specific interactions. In order to fully grasp the manifestation of insight observed in this clinical interaction, then, it is essential to first outline the general features and constraints of clinical interactions.

Since the 1950s, there has been an increasing interest in examining the doctor-patient relationship from a number of perspectives. Heritage and Maynard (2006, 2) highlight Charon *et al.*'s assertion that doctor-patient interaction has more recently been studied from one of two perspectives: microanalysis of discourse and process analysis. The present chapter draws upon the tools of microanalysis of discourse within doctor-patient communication. Heritage and Maynard (2006, 2–6) provide a historical overview of the work that has been done in this area, beginning with Byrne and Long's groundbreaking 1976 work *Doctors Talking to Patients*. As the title of this work suggests, much of the previous work that was done in this field focused primarily on the doctor (e.g., Roter *et al.*'s [1997] *Communication Patterns of Primary Care Physicians;* Beckman and Frankel's [1984] *The Effect of Physician Behavior on the Collection of Data*). More recently, doctor-patient interaction research has focused on the co-construction of the clinical visit. As ten Have (2005, 138) discusses, mainly in relation to acute care visits, "medical encounters display a rather conventional organization in terms of phases devoted to specific consecutive tasks in the encounter…But, on a more detailed level, this overall organization has to be realized through series of concerted activities that are sequentially organized" by both physicians and patients.

Much of the previous research on the microanalysis of discourse within medical interactions has focused on primary-care and acute medical visits, analyzing the sequential organization of their different phases (e.g., problem

presentation, history-taking, diagnosis, treatment recommendation, and closing (Robinson and Heritage 2005, 481). The clinical interaction analyzed in
this paper, however, is routine; routine visits often lack the defined structure
of an acute care visit (Heritage, personal communication, August 8, 2008). In
this chapter's focal interaction, the patient sees her doctor every three to six
months for routine follow-up visits: almost the entire interaction is comprised
of history-taking. Within the clinic, it is expected that the only topic and
focus will be the patient and his/her concerns. In this way, the clinic is an ideal
environment in which to explore issues of self and insight for FTD patients.

During the clinical interview with an FTD patient to be shown in the examples that follow, authority regarding oneself is problematized because of
the patient's unawareness of certain issues related to her condition. In many
cases, the patient invokes her daughter, the caregiver, as an authority on problems she herself may be experiencing. In her research on clinical interactions
involving three parties (physician, patient, and parent), Stivers (2001, 253)
notes, "the presence of a third party has already been shown in the existing
literature to significantly affect the interaction (e.g., Lerner 1993; Sacks *et al.*
1974; Schegloff 1995; Simmel, 1950)." For example, she observes, "in the
course of the interaction, the parent and the child may be treated both as a
single party and as two parties" (Stivers 2001, 253). In addition, the triadic
dynamic found in interactions with FTD patients is similar to clinical interactions involving children with chronic illness and their parents (Clemente
*et al.* 2008) in that clinicians elicit information from the patient but the patient
frequently involves his/her caregiver through inviting corroboration or confirmation of responses. In this way, in the examples that form this case study, the
"self" seems to be distributed over both the patient and her caregiver.

### Question-response Sequences

As described above, in addition to questionnaires, neurologists often use general or open-ended questioning to determine the patient's level of insight.
The design of questions, however, can often carry presuppositions about the
participants. Indeed, as Heritage (2002a, 314) emphasizes, "regardless of the
specific aims of the question, the ways in which questions are designed unavoidably serve to index the relationship between questioner and respondent."
Physicians' questions often work to select and constrain patients' responses
before they are even given. This is a crucial element in this chapter's focal
interaction, as the patient listens to and utilizes the questions' placement,
design, and content as resources in forming responses. To adequately analyze
the patient's display of insight through her responses, it is necessary to preserve their place in sequences of talk and specifically in relation to the physician's questions. In conversation analytic literature, there has been a large

body of work devoted to question design and question-response sequences in both naturally-occurring and institutional settings such as clinical interactions. The following sections will highlight aspects of this body of work that are most relevant to the present data analysis.

### Question and Response Design

In their discussion of history-taking during the medical visit, Boyd and Heritage (2006, 154–163) highlight the fact that question design both conveys and solicits information, exemplified by some of the following characteristics and shown in Table 5.2 below. They note that questions set agendas, embody presuppositions, and incorporate preferences. Questions can set topic agendas; they foreground certain issues as topics of inquiry. They can also set action agendas by asking a recipient to give substantial information, clarify, and justify. Questions embody the principle of recipient design, a term that refers to the way in which speakers design their talk to display "an orientation and sensitivity to the particular other(s) who are the coparticipants" (Sacks *et al.* 1974, 727). In this data, question design is particularly relevant since the doctor relies on the patient's responses in order to build an understanding of the patient's experience.

A response is a general category which includes answers. Clayman and Heritage (2002, 242) define an answer as "an action that addresses the agenda of topics and tasks posed by a previous question." As will become evident through an analysis of this data, the patient's responses do not always conform to the action and/or topic agendas of the questions posed to them. Thus their responses are not always "answers." In addition, the patient's responses may or may not confirm the doctor's presuppositions or align with his preferences (discussed in the following section). At times, the doctor may take this range of non-aligning behavior as evidence for the lack of insight the patient has about her own condition.

### Preference Structure

As Atkinson and Heritage (1984, 53) discuss, "the concept of 'preference' has developed in conversation analytic research to characterize conversational

| **Physician Questions** | **Patient Responses** |
|---|---|
| Set Agendas:<br>(i) Topical agendas<br>(ii) Action agendas | Engage/Decline to engage:<br>(i) Topical agendas<br>(ii) Action agendas |
| Embody presuppositions | Confirm/Disconfirm presuppositions |
| Incorporate preferences | Align/Disalign with preferences |

Table 5.2   Dimensions of Questioning and Answering

events in which alternative, but nonequivalent, courses of action are available to the participants (Sacks 1973). [These] alternatives may arise at the level of lexical selection, utterance design, and action or sequence choice." Preference structure plays an integral part in the design of the doctor's questions and, in turn, the responses the patient gives.

## The Interactive Nature of Questioning and Responding in the Medical Setting

Based on much the information highlighted in the previous sections, Heritage (2010, 45) models the various dimensions of questioning and responding in medical encounters (Table 5.2 opposite, which is also included in Boyd and Heritage [2006]). This table emphasizes the interactive nature of questioning and responding in the medical setting, as physician and patient mutually shape each other's next turns throughout the interaction.

Heritage (2010, 42) emphasizes medical educator Eric Cassell's notion that "during history taking, the physician may seek to become 'a fixed measuring instrument,' a kind of living questionnaire, neutral and consistent across patients (1985, 89). In pursuit of this objective, however, clinicians will not adopt the style of questioning to be found in social surveys and other kinds of 'fixed measuring instruments' (Heritage 2002a)." Heritage (2010, 43–44) highlights the centrality of question design within the clinical interaction: "To be effective, physicians…must build questions that instantiate a caring relationship with patients. The primary means by which they can do this is 'recipient design'… (Sacks *et al.* 1974, 727). The consequence of recipient design in the medical context is not only a departure from 'neutral' questioning but also, associated with this, the communication of the physician's reasoning, beliefs, and expectations. Thus, as Cassell (1985, 4) also notes, 'Even when we physicians ask questions, the structure of the questions and their wording provides information about ourselves, our intent, our beliefs about patients and diseases, as well as eliciting such information about patients; 'taking a history' is unavoidably and actually an *exchange* of information' (italics in the original)."

The present analysis will examine this interactive "exchange" as it manifests itself across sequences during the clinical interview. In this way, it will illuminate both how through their questions doctors attempt to locate patient's insight and how patients may or may not demonstrate that they have it through their responses during the clinical interview.

## Study Design

This research is a case study, based on video-taped data of a routine clinical visit collected at a neurology clinic. The patient's name is Louise; at the time of the taping she was 70 years old. The focal interaction was a regular checkup, and included the doctor (DOCT), patient (LOIS), and her caregiver daughter (JESS). Data analysis will draw upon the methods and tools of conversation analysis (Sacks *et al.* 1974). The clinical data analyzed here is intended to complement the Social Relations in FTD Research Group data collected in naturally-occurring interactions in patients' homes and others settings. Focusing on the details of one clinical visit makes it possible to highlight both the routinized conversational practices employed by the doctor in addition to the specific contingencies of this interaction and patient.

## Insight and Conversational Practices in the Clinic

As described above, in an effort to identify features of insight in the clinic, the following analysis will focus on the details and contingencies of question-response sequences. More specifically, it will highlight some of the clinician's conversational practices, presuppositions, and aims in his exploration of the patient's insight. It will also demonstrate how the patient's responses frequently exhibit resistance to the doctor's presuppositions and preference structures as exhibited in his question design, in addition to emphasizing how the patient involves her caregiver as a resource in order to respond to these questions.

In Example 5.2 the doctor's question design begins with certain presuppositions and then shifts in response to the patient's responses. Over the course of the interaction, there is a gradual shift in the order of business as the questions become more focused. At the beginning, the doctor is interested in whether or not the patient has experienced problems, but over time he becomes more actively interested in whether the patient has specific problems. As the following analysis will demonstrate, his transition into questions focused on the specificity of the patient's problems is both contingent on and influential in her demonstrations of certain kinds of insight. (Please see Appendix B for transcription notations.)

The doctor's turn at line 12, *Tell me what kind of problems you're having*, is presuppositionally loaded for a description of the patient's problems. In other words, by designing his turn in this way, the doctor is presupposing that the patient has problems since the preferred next response would be Louise then describing her problems. Since this is a routine visit, this presupposition is most likely based on previous visits with this patient and/or caregiver reports. Robinson (2006, 36), in a consideration of how doctors solicit patients' presenting concerns, notes that there are certain question formats that are "designed to index chronic-routine visits." Some examples are "What's new?" or "Anything new?" (Robinson 2006, 36–37). In this way then, the doctor's first pair part at line 12 is distinctive among chronic-routine visits because it does not orient to the possibility of these problems being new. The doctor's utterance at line 12 does however exhibit a presupposition that she has problems, since he does not ask *if* she has any problems and instead asks

```
5.2 Problems Not at All
Louise Clinic Visit

01   DOCT    Okay well lemme ask you some questions uh- (0.5) Mrs.
02           Peterson uh-
03   LOIS    You're gonna have to talk louder.
04   DOCT    Lemme ask you uh- s- lemme ask you some [questions.]
05   LOIS                                           [How come ] I
06           didn't wear my hearing aids? ((turns to Jess))
07   JESS    They're not working properly.
08   LOIS    Well the ears aren't either.
09           (3.0)
10   DOCT    [Uh:]
11   JESS    [I'd] take your ears off if I could as wellhhhh.
12   DOCT    Tell me what kind of problems you're having.
13   LOIS    Problems?
14   DOCT    ((nods head slightly))
15   LOIS    Not at all.
16   DOCT    No problems?
17   LOIS    No.
18           (1.0)
19   LOIS    Not that I can think of anything serious.
20   DOCT    Do you have any difficulties? Uh- any memory problems
21           or speaking problems or (0.2) any- [any problems?]
22   LOIS                                       [I think I'm  ]
23           (about) the same as I always have been ((turns to
24           Jess)) right?
25   JESS    You're y'know you're you forget things.
26   LOIS    Yeah. [But it doesn't bother me.]
27   JESS          [And sometimes you get    ] confused over ti:me
28           and- and- like this morning she thought that her watch
29           had stopped and she was still on Florida time.
30   LOIS    Oh man. Why don't I have my hearing aids in.
31   JESS    'Cause we didn't put them in because they're not
32           working right. We have to get them fixed.
33   LOIS    Because I forgot them. Hehehehehehehehe.
```

her *what kind* of problems she is having.

At line 13, the patient initiates repair with *Problems?*. Repair has been defined by Schegloff (2000, 207) as orderly "practices for dealing with problems or troubles in speaking, hearing, and understanding the talk in conversation." As Bolden (2009, 121) has described, turn constructional units such as *Problems?* are termed repeat prefacing and are "used by conversationalists to resist agendas and presuppositions generated by questions and other sequence initiating actions." By repeating a lexical item used in the previous term, the patient's other-initiated repair is in contrast to Drew's (1997, 73) classification of open-class repair initiators such as "Pardon" or "Sorry." Open-class repair initiators "offer no explicit account of the nature of the trouble which the speaker might be having; nor do they give any indication of specifically what it is in, or about, the prior turn that is causing difficulty." In contrast, in her response the patient locates precisely what the trouble source is and thus indexes the issues she has with the notion embodied in the doctor's question. Her next turn constructional unit (TCU) at line 15, *Not at all.*, is a decisive response that reveals the fact that she does not believe she has any problems. Here then, it is evident how the patient pushes back against the doctor's presupposition as embodied in his question design at line 12.

At line 16, the doctor reopens his line of inquiry, not allowing progressivity (see Mikesell, Chapter 4, this volume) through his reformulation of the previous question (*No problems?*). This question, which provides the patient with a chance to revise her previous response, seeks confirmation as its polarity is tilted towards a "yes" response. His maintenance of this line of questioning may index the central relevance of insight at this point. The patient then provides a reconfirmation of her previous decisive response at lines 17–19 (*No. (1.0) Not that I can think of anything serious.*). What is important to note here is that she now re-does her previous response, providing a qualification (*Not that I can think of anything serious.*). A qualification of this type may indeed demonstrate a degree of insight, in that the patient is considering the problems she might have and their seriousness in her life.

After this 4-line sequence (lines 16–19), the doctor shifts his question design to include three instances of the negative polarity item *any* (lines 20–21). Negative polarity items such as "any" and "at all" used in questions establish a "practice-based preference (Schegloff 1988) for a *No*-type response" (Robinson 2006, 6). By using negative polarity items in his turn, the doctor is building his questions for a specific type of response. He begins with a general class that is more explicit than *problems* (*difficulties*), moves to more specific types of problems (*memory problems, speaking problems*), and completes his three-part list (Jefferson 1990) with a move back to a general class (*problems*). Therefore, due to the patient's responses, the doctor shifts his turn and question design from those that presuppose that she has problems to those that are tilted toward "no" responses. He thus moves to a question design that pushes her to think of any examples of problems, which now incorporates elements that are pushing toward an expected "no" response. In this way, one can begin to note the reciprocal nature of this interaction, where questions affect next responses and responses affect next questions.

In response to the doctor's questions at lines 20 and 21, the patient says *I think I'm the same as I always have been ([turns to Jess]) right?*. First, she uses the epistemic marker *think*, which signals a form of downgraded epistemics, especially since she is using it in reference to her own experience. She then construes her response in terms of her past self in comparison with her present state. In this way, she is orienting both to the regular nature of such visits and to the fact that the visit is routine and not motivated by any specific problems. Until this point, the interaction has included only the doctor and the patient, though the caregiver has been in the room. By shifting her gaze towards her caregiver and requesting confirmation with *right?*, the patient invites corroboration. She thus acknowledges the fact that she may not have the complete answer; her response is indexical of the notion that another party could know better than she does. At line 25 she then confirms what Jess says with *Yeah. But it doesn't bother me.* In addition, her utterance at line 32 (*Because I forgot them.*) exhibits a level of insight, for she has now jokingly incorporated the information her daughter had provided at line 24.

The patient's various actions in this excerpt may not exhibit evidence of the current self-focused definition of insight. However, they do potentially demonstrate a different level of insight, one which involves the patient's knowledge about someone else's knowledge state. The patient exhibits a movement towards incorporating others' input into defining her condition. This excerpt highlights the fact that the patient does have a version of herself, and that she verifies whether others may have a different version of her than she does.

The patient deploys similar resources in Example 5.3, shown below. In this example, the doctor again asks if the patient has any problems, this time with starting a project and finishing it. Her response is delayed after 2.0 seconds, but she eventually provides an unequivocal *No. I get a project I'll do it.* But, then, after 0.5 seconds, she again turns to her caregiver so that she may provide corroboration of the information the patient has just provided. Again, she seems to be exhibiting an awareness of the fact that someone else may have a different version of her than she does, demonstrating insight into the potential relevance of others' opinions.

In Example 5.4 below, which follows directly after line 33 of Example 5.2, one can observe similar patterns to those highlighted in the previous excerpts. In Example 5.2, the doctor shifts from an utterance design that presupposes

```
5.3 Get a Project
Louise Clinic Visit


01   DOCT    Do you have uh- any problems say uh- with uh- (0.3) uh
02           starting a project and finishing it.
03           (2.0)
04   LOIS    No. I get a project I'll do it.
05           (0.5)
06   LOIS    Right? ((turns to Jess))
07   JESS    Yes if I give you a project you will do it initiating
08           the project is another issue. Only thing she initiates
09           is reading the paper [or reading:g            ]=
10   LOIS                         [Is he taking my picture?]
11   JESS    =books. She'll start that.
12           (3.0)
13   DOCT    I see. What kinda books do you read?
```

```
5.4 Not Past Past But
Louise Clinic Visit

01   DOCT    So do you think you have a memory problem?
02   LOIS    Oh yeah.
03           (3.0)
04   DOCT    How bad is it?
05   LOIS    But I remember you.
06           (2.0)
07   LOIS    Now that I see you. Before I didn't.
08           (3.0)
09   DOCT    Oh:. So you remember that you didn't remember me.
10   LOIS    ((shrugs))
11   DOCT    Hehehe.
12   JESS    That's a plus.
13   LOIS    I didn't remember what you look like.
14           (0.5)
15   DOCT    So uh do you think uh your memory problem is ah- (0.2)
16           is it significant for you
17   LOIS    (Eh)
18   DOCT    Hm?
19   LOIS    Doesn't bother me.
20   DOCT    It doesn't bother you. What kinds of things uh- give you
21           a problem remembering?
22           (6.0)
23   LOIS    Not past past (0.2) but (0.2) um-
24           (3.0)
25   LOIS    ((looks at caregiver))
26   JESS    Recent past.
27   LOIS    [Yeah. Recent past.]
28   JESS    [You're correct.    ]
```

the patient has problems to one that is tilted toward "no" responses. In line 1
of example 5.4, the doctor's question design shifts to incorporate the use of
the epistemic marker *think* (which the patient uses earlier at line 22 of example 5.2). This turn design downgrades the patient's right to know the information. Ordinarily, a person has absolute rights over subjective experience.
But, in this context, her apprehension of subjective experience is exactly what
is at issue. The question "So do you think you have a memory problem?" may
qualify or downgrade the patient's rights to know the information, given that
the ordinary form is "Do you have a memory problem?" (Heritage, personal
communication, October 29, 2009).[1]

The patient's response at line 2 is an oh-prefaced response to an inquiry
(Heritage 1998). Heritage (1998, 291) notes that "in responses to English

---

1.  It is interesting to note that at line 1 of Example 5.4 the "Do you think" formulation undermines the patient's right to know, while normally such a formulation would invite an
    opinion statement and thus privilege the patient's authority over her own experience. A
    memory problem is something that one would know about oneself, but in this case the question formulation downgrades the patient's authority over reporting on her own experience.

questions, prefacing with the particle *oh* indicates that, from the viewpoint of the answerer, a question is problematic in terms of its relevance, presuppositions, or context. In addition, oh-prefacing is used to foreshadow reluctance to advance the conversational topic invoked by a question." In this case, through her response the patient asserts her epistemic authority and indexes the fact that the answer is obvious. In line 5 *But I remember you,* the patient asserts what she *is* able to do.

At lines 15 and 16, the doctor struggles in framing his next question, as evidenced by a number of restarts and self-repairs (*So uh do you think uh your memory problem is ah- (0.2) is it significant for you?*). The various versions of the question that he begins with index the epistemics of understanding a memory problem. A memory problem, though experienced by one person, is something which is intersubjectively visible to others (Heritage, personal communication, August 8, 2008). The question design that the doctor finally uses, *is it significant for you?*, subjectivizes the memory problem and invites an opinion statement about it on the part of the patient. By repairing his utterance and ending with this turn design, he is able to ask the patient a question about something which she has exclusive and primary rights to know. Whether or not her memory problem is significant for her is something that others would not be able to speak to. The patient then provides a response at line 19 that expresses the fact that her memory problem is not significant for her.

In response to the doctor's question at lines 20 and 21, the patient waits six seconds before responding. At line 23, she articulates her memory problem as *not past past but um.* She frames the word search as a contrast, and during a three second pause she scrunches her face and looks at her caregiver. In so doing, the patient displays forgetfulness and thus provides a "[resource] for emerging interaction" (Goodwin 1987, 116). At line 26, Jess completes the patient's utterance with *recent past,* thus creating a collaboratively complete utterance (Sacks 1992; Lerner 1991). At line 27, the patient corroborates the completion of her utterance with *Yeah.* In her next turn constructional unit she then corroborates and owns the information by repeating what her caregiver said, *Recent past.* Lastly, Jess assesses the previously co-constructed utterance with *You're correct.* (line 28). By addressing her mother with *you* and producing an assessment, Jess casts the utterance as something which her mother now has ownership of and which is then assessable by others.

In both excerpts 5.2 and 5.4, the doctor asks questions that embody certain presuppositions. The patient responds in ways that do not conform to these presuppositions or she equivocates in some way. At the invitation of the patient, the caregiver then provides responses that conform more expressly to the doctor's original presuppositions as embodied in his question design. Interestingly, in a clinical assessment given to Louise without her daughter in the room (after the examples discussed in this chapter), Louise states, "I'm lucky I have my daughters." Louise herself recognizes the importance of having her daughter present so that they can collaboratively provide the information the doctor is seeking. The doctor asks a number of questions, which provides the patient with the opportunity to display both what she is aware of and that she is aware of others' versions of herself. In both of these examples, insight manifests itself interactionally as something distributed over more than one speaker.

In the next Example 5.5, which occurs approximately six minutes after the previous example, the doctor begins a line of questions focused on changes the patient may have experienced in recent years. At line 1, the doctor's questions orient toward changes the patient may have experienced, beginning (as he did in Example 5.1) with general questions (e.g., *Have you changed...*, *Are you different...*). The patient responds at line 4 with *Not that I'm aware of.* This response embodies great carefulness, as the patient acknowledges that there are some things she can assert and other things that she cannot. She recognizes that it is possible that she would not know about some changes, and that there could be a problem that she would not be aware of. At lines 5–6, 9, and 11–12, the doctor moves toward more specific possibilities (e.g., *political affiliation, religion, philosophy*). In some cases, it has been shown that FTD patients have had drastic changes in such belief systems (Miller *et al.* 2001), which is most likely driving this line of inquiry. Here again, the patient utters an oh-prefaced response at line 13 (*Oh no:.*), which embodies the fact that the doctor's previous question was "problematic in terms of its relevance, presuppositions, or context" (Heritage 1998, 291).

At lines 16 and 17, the doctor then moves to another general question (*An uh- (.) in general do you see yourself as different now than you were ten years ago?*). This is another attempt to ascertain her insight about changes in her personality and preferences. After the patient's repair initiator at line 18 (*Do I seem different?*), the doctor redoes his question (*Do you see your*self *as different now*), which highlights that he is asking about *her* version of herself. The grammatical design of the question invites a "yes" response. But at line 21, the patient confidently responds with a flat-out refusal (*No. No. I don't.*). However, after a 0.3 second silence, she displays her recognition that her daughter might see her as different (*Maybe they do.*). She then turns to her caregiver, addressing her and asking *Do you see me as different?*. Though this question (one of the only questions that the patient asks in the entire interaction that is not a repair initiator) is yes-preferring, there is still the overhang of her *No. No. I don't.* response from line 21. Finally, Jess's humorous utterance response at line 25 is somewhat responsive to Louise's question. In this last example, it is evident that though the patient may not recognize changes in herself, she does acknowledge the fact that her daughter may see her differently.

```
5.5 See Me as Different
Louise Clinic Visit

01  DOCT    U:m: have you changed over the last uh- (0.5) few
02          years? Have- Are you- are you different in en- um your
03          preferences and attitudes en-
04  LOIS    Not that I'm aware of.
05  DOCT    Political affiliation. Religion. [Any  ] of those
06          things.
07  LOIS                                     [What?]
08  LOIS    Ability?
09  DOCT    Have you changed ina- your philosophy er-
10          (0.4)
11  DOCT    Er in your yaknow your politics or your religious
12          beliefs er-
13  LOIS    Oh no:.
14  DOCT    S'all been the same.
15  LOIS    ((Nods head)) Yeah.
16  DOCT    And uh- (.) in general do you see yourself as
17          different now than you were ten years ago?
18  LOIS    Do I seem different?
19  DOCT    Do you see yourself as different
20          n[ow than ten years ago?]
21  LOIS     [No. I don't.          ]
22          (0.3)
23  LOIS    Maybe they do. ((turns to Jess)) Do you see me as
24          different?
25  JESS    I see you more often but not as different[hehehehehe.]
26  DOCT                                             [Hehehehehe.]
```

## Converging Evidence with Other Data Collection Methods

The research presented here complements some of the information found when doctors at UCLA Medical Center gave patients the "UCLA FTD Insight Scale." Patients were able to respond appropriately to questions 5–8, but less so to questions 1–4 (Mendez, personal communication, May 15, 2008). In other words, patients recognized that other people are aware of or are concerned about their personality changes and the disease, although they themselves may not demonstrate a recognition of this problem on their own.

**UCLA FTD Insight Scale** (results reported in Mendez and Shapira 2005):

1. Do you have an illness or problem that requires medical attention?

2. How concerned are you about your illness/problem?

3. Is your behavior/personality significantly different now, compared to a few years ago?

4. How concerned are you about your behavioral/personality change?

5. Do family/friends think that you have an illness or problem that requires medical attention?

6. How concerned are you that family/friends worry about your illness/problem?

7. Do family/friends think that you have had a behavior change, compared to a few years ago?

8. How concerned are you that family/friends worry about your behavior change?

This research, then, is able to provide a detailed complement to the information gained through questionnaires such as the UCLA FTD Insight Scale. Through an in-depth analysis of insight in interaction, one is able to grasp how patients may or may not utilize caregivers as resources in the clinic. This case study has highlighted the distributed and interactive aspects of insight as it manifests itself during clinical interviews.

## Implications

In the above examples, Louise was consistently encouraged to articulate information about her problems and concerns. Though in general she did not at first acknowledge that she has problems, upon more questioning, she moved towards incorporating her daughter's version of her condition. She was thus exhibiting a different kind of insight, in which she was able to recognize that others may have different knowledge or information about her and her mental state. The patient did have a version of herself, but she consistently involved her caregiver so that the caregiver could provide information to augment or complement this. The patient's involvement of her caregiver was a mechanism that provided *another* version, one that in many cases conformed more tightly to the doctor's presuppositions or preference structure as embodied in his question design.

During naturally-occurring interactions in the home and other settings, such as those discussed in other chapters in this volume, patients are not generally asked questions about what they are or are not aware of.[2] But, the clinic's focus on the patient provides a unique interactional setting in which to explore

---

2. However, in the following naturally-occurring interaction, the issue of Louise's awareness of her condition does surface. Here, she seems to exhibit concern about her condition as she introduces a question about whether she acts differently from "the norm". This example includes Louise (LOIS), her daughter Jess (JESS), her daughter Dana (DANA), and Michael (MICH), as they are driving home from going out for a meal and shopping. In this example outside of the clinic, Louise does demonstrate an awareness of her condition, though based on a dependence on others' perceptions. She seeks to confirm the presence of an illness by asking Mick the question at line 01. In addition, through her use of *supposedly* in line 9, she is questioning what others have told her about herself.

issues of self and insight. In Louise's case, the doctor's sequential pursuit of insight through a number of general and specific questions provided the patient with the opportunity to demonstrate what types of insight she does have. She was able to accomplish this through her articulation of her own perspectives in addition to the use of additional interactional resources such as her daughter. In this way, it became possible to see the more complex demonstrations of insight over the course of the institutional interaction. If the issue of insight had not been pursued by the doctor, she would not have had the opportunity to exhibit this distributed insight. In this example, then, it became possible for a more complex picture of insight to manifest itself sequentially.

What is striking here is that in the previously analyzed examples, it was not necessary to administer a test to Louise in order to gauge her ability to recognize others' mental states. In fact, during naturally-occurring interactions during the clinical interview she consistently invited and incorporated her daughter's perspective as a means of corroborating/triangulating the evidence she may have been presenting. This was a thorough and detailed display of both insight and Theory of Mind, for it demonstrated her consistent attempt to create a co-constructed and accurate representation of her symptoms (Heritage, personal communication, April 24, 2009). Previous ToM measures consider the patient in isolation, taking tests about imaginary people and situations with which the patient is not previously familiar. The evidence presented here demonstrates that perhaps more ecological and effective tests of Theory of Mind would include more personally relevant information in addition to the involvement of one's caregiver. In addition, by providing patients with naturally-occurring opportunities to demonstrate Theory of Mind, clinicians may be able to ascertain other features of the disease that are not evident through current clinical measures.

The present analysis reveals that insight includes both an awareness of one's problems and a recognition that one could have problems that one is unaware of. Therefore, insight is a multi-faceted concept that individuals do not

```
5.6 Act Differently
Louise Car Ride


01   LOIS     <Do:: I: a:::ct> (0.4) differently?
02   MICH     Do you act differen[tly?]
03   LOIS                        [Yeah]
04   MICH     Then what?
05   LOIS     From the norm?
06   MICH     From the norm?
07   LOIS     Yeah
08   MICH     No not really
09   LOIS     Because I have I- I supposedly have this fronta tempura
10            thing
11   MICH     Uh huh
12   KATE     Tempura thing heh heh heh heh
```

simply have or lack. Instead, there may be something closer to an "insight continuum," which patients would find themselves on at different stages of the disease. Clinicians' recognition of a more complex picture of insight could potentially help to distinguish different stages of the disease. In addition, it demonstrates the interdependence of many diagnostic features of the disease, including insight and social and interpersonal conduct. This analysis also highlights the importance of having copresent caregivers during clinical interactions, such that patients would have the ability to utilize them as resources during clinical interviews.

This case study provides valuable information about the conversational practices routinely used by the doctor to determine whether or not a patient has insight. It also reveals that this specific patient is able to exhibit certain kinds of insight, though these may or may not match the current clinical definitions of this phenomenon. The interactional focus presented in this research suggests that insight, as an observable feature of FTD, is more than something that resides in the brain of one individual. Instead, it is something that manifests itself interactionally among copresent interlocutors. This analysis demonstrates that the notion of insight as it is used as a diagnostic criterion for FTD should in fact include a component in which the individual recognizes that there are problems or issues he or she may not be aware of, that others may have more knowledge or information about. By recognizing that this type of insight is possible, doctors may pursue the issue beyond a sequence of two to three questions as seen in Example 5.1. In so doing, they may discover aspects of patients' insight that until this point may have been concealed.

## References

Atkinson, J.M. and Heritage, J. (eds.)

1984 *Structures of Social Action: Studies in Conversation Analysis*. Cambridge: Cambridge University Press.

Beckman, H. and Frankel, R.

1984 The effect of physician behavior on the collection of data. *Annals of Internal Medicine* 101: 692–696.

Bolden, G.

2009 Beyond answering: Repeat-prefaced responses in conversation. *Communication Monographs* 76(2): 121–143.

Boyd, J.H.

2008 Have We Found the Holy Grail? Theory of Mind as a Unifying Construct. *Journal of Religion and Health* 47: 366–385.

Boyd, E. and J. Heritage.

2006 Taking the Patient's Medical History: Questioning During Comprehensive History Taking. In *Communication in Medical Care: Interactions between Primary Care Physicians and Patients,* edited by J. Heritage and D. Maynard, 151–184. Cambridge: Cambridge University Press.

Byrne, P.S. and B.E.L. Long.

1976 *Doctors Talking to Patients: A Study of the Verbal Behaviours of Doctors in the Consultation.* London: Her Majesty's Stationery Office.

Cassell, E.

1985 *Talking with Patients, Volume 2: Clinical Technique.* Cambridge, MA: MIT Press.

Charon, R., M.J. Greene and R. Adelman.

1994 Multidimensional interaction analysis: a collaborative approach to the study of medical discourse. *Social Science and Medicine* 39(7): 955–965.

Clemente, I., S. Lee and J. Heritage.

2008 Children in chronic pain: Promoting pediatric patients' symptom accounts in tertiary care. *Social Science and Medicine* 66(6): 1418–1428.

Clayman, S. and J. Heritage.

2002 *The News Interview: Journalists and Public Figures on the Air.* Cambridge: Cambridge University Press.

Drew, P.

1997 'Open' class repair initiators in response to sequential sources of troubles in conversation. *Journal of Pragmatics* 28(1): 69–101.

Eslinger, P.J., P. Moore, V. Trolani, S. Antani, K. Cross, S. Kwok and M. Grossman

2007 Oops! Resolving social dilemmas in frontotemporal dementia. *Journal of Neurology, Neurosurgery, and Psychiatry* 78: 457–460.

Evers, K., L. Kilander and M. Lindau.

2007 Insight in frontotemporal dementia: Conceptual analysis and empirical evaluation of the consensus criterion "loss of insight" in frontotemporal dementia. *Brain and Cognition* 63: 13–23.

Fernandez-Duque, D., Baird, J.A., and Black, S.E.

2009 False-belief understanding in fronto-temporal dementia and Alzheimer's disease. *Journal of Clinical and Experimental Neuropsychology* 31(4): 489–497.

Goodwin, C.

1987 Forgetfulness as an interactive resource. *Social Psychology Quarterly* 50: 115–130.

Gregory, C., S. Lough, V. Stone, S. Erzinclioglu, L. Martin, S. Baron-Cohen and J.R. Hodges

2002 Theory of mind in patients with frontal variant frontotemporal dementia and Alzheimer's disease: Theoretical and practical implications. *Brain* 125: 752–764.

Heritage, J.

1998 Oh-prefaced Responses to Inquiry. *Language in Society* 27(3): 291–334.

2002a Ad hoc inquiries: two preferences in the design of 'routine' questions in an open context. In *Standardization and Tacit Knowledge: Interaction and Practice in the Survey Interview*, edited by D. Maynard, H. Houtkoop-Steenstra, N.K. Schaeffer and  H. van der Zouwen, 313–333. New York: Wiley Interscience.

2002b The Limits of Questioning: Negative Interrogatives and Hostile Question Content. *Journal of Pragmatics* 34: 1427–1446.

2010 Questioning in Medicine. In *"Why Do You Ask?": The Function of Questions in Institutional Discourse*, edited by A. Freed and S. Ehrlich, 42–68. New York: Oxford University Press.

Heritage, J. and D. Maynard.

2006 *Communication in Medical Care: Interaction Between Primary Care Physicians and Patients*. Cambridge: Cambridge University Press.

Jefferson, G.

1990 List-Construction as a Task and Resource. In *Interactional competence.* edited by G. Psathas, 63–92. New York: Irvington Publishers.

Kipps, C.M. and J.R. Hodges

2006 Theory of mind in frontotemporal dementia. *Social Neuroscience* 1(3): 235–244.

Lerner, G.

1991 On the syntax of sentences-in-progress. *Language in Society* 20: 441–458.

1993 Collectivities in action: Establishing the relevance of conjoined participation in conversation. *Text* 13(2): 213–245.

Lough, S., C.M. Kipps, C. Treise, P. Watson, J.R. Blair and J.R. Hodges

2006 Social reasoning, emotion and empathy in frontotemporal dementia. *Neuropsychologia* 44: 950–958.

Mendez, M.F. and J. Shapira.

2005 Loss of Insight and Functional Neuroimaging in Frontotemporal Dementia. *Journal of Neurospychiatry and Clinical Neurosciences* 17: 413–416.

Miller, B.L., W.W. Seeley, P. Mychack, H. J. Rosen, I. Mena and K. Boone.

2001 Neuroanatomy of the self: Evidence from patients with frontotemporal dementia. *Neurology* 57(5): 817–821.

Neary D, J.S. Snowden, L. Gustafson, U. Passant, D. Stuss and S. Black.

1998 Frontotemporal lobar degeneration: A consensus on clinical diagnostic criteria. *Neurology* 51: 1546–1554.

Neary D., J.S. Snowden and D.M.A. Mann.

2005 Frontotemporal dementia. *Lancet Neurology* 4: 771–779.

O'Keeffe, F.M., B. Murray, R.F. Coen, P.M. Dockree, M.A. Bellgrove, H. Garavan, T. Lynch and I.H. Robertson.

2007 Loss of insight in frontotemporal dementia, corticobasal degeneration and progressive supranuclear palsy. *Brain*. 130: 753–764.

Rabins, P.V., C.G. Lyketsos and C. Steele.

2006 *Practical dementia care*. Oxford University Press.

Rankin, K.P., E. Baldwin, C. Pace-Savitsky, J.H. Kramer and B.L. Miller.

2005 Self awareness and personality change in dementia. *Journal of Neurology, Neurosurgery, and Psychiatry* 76: 632–639.

Robinson, J.D.

2006 Soliciting patients' presenting concerns. In *Communication in Medical Care: Interactions between Primary Care Physicians and Patients,* edited by J. Heritage and D. Maynard, 23–47. Cambridge: Cambridge University Press.

Robinson, J.D. and J. Heritage.

2005 The Structure of Patients' Presenting Concerns: The Completion Relevance of Current Symptoms. *Social Science and Medicine* 61(2): 481–493.

Roter, D., M. Stewart, S. Putnam, M. Lipkin, W. Stiles and T.S. Inui.

1997 Communication patterns of primary care physicians. *Journal of the American Medical Association* 227(4): 350–6.

Sacks, H.

1973 The preference for agreement in natural conversation. Paper presented at the Linguistic Institute. Ann Arbor, Michigan.
1992 [1967-1968] In Lectures on Conversation, vols. I and II, edited by G. Jefferson, xx-xx. Oxford: Blackwell Publishing

Sacks, H., E.A. Schegloff and G. Jefferson.

1974 A Simplest Systematics for the Organization of Turn-Taking for Conversation. *Language* 50(4): 696–735.

Salmon, E., D. Perani, F. Collette, D. Feyers, E. Kalbe, V. Holthoff, S. Sorbi and K. Herholz.

2008 A comparison of unawareness in frontotemporal dementia and Alzheimer's disease. *Journal of Neurology, Neurosurgery, and Psychiatry* 79: 176–179.

Schegloff, E.A.

1988 On an Actual Virtual Servo-Mechanism for Guessing Bad News: A Single Case Conjecture. *Social Problems* 35: 442–457.

1995 Parties and Talking Together: Two Ways in Which Numbers Are Significant for Talk-in-Interaction. In *Situated Order: Studies in Social Organization and Embodied Activities,* edited by P. ten Have and G. Psathas, 31–42. Washington, DC: University Press of America.

2000 When 'Others' Initiate Repair. *Applied Linguistics* 21(2): 205–243.

Simmel, G.

1950 *The sociology of Georg Simmel.* Translated by Kurt Wolff. Glencoe, IL: Free Press.

Stivers, T.

2001 Negotiating Who Presents the Problem: Next Speaker Selection in Pediatric Encounters. *Journal of Communication* 51(2): 252–282.

ten Have, P.

2005 Talk and Institution: A Reconsideration of the "Asymmetry of Doctor-Patient Interaction. In *Talk and Social Structure: Studies in Ethnomethodology and Conversation Analysis,* 138–163. Berkeley: University of California Press.

$$— 6 —$$

# Using Social Deficits in Frontotemporal Dementia to Develop a Neurobiology of Person Reference

Andrea W. Mates

Many of us have fond, and sometimes embarrassing, memories of reviewing family photographs and introducing people, events, and locations of personal significance to others. I had the opportunity, on my second participant-observation ethnography visit with a 62 year old frontotemporal dementia (FTD) patient "Romeo", to look over some of his photographs with him as we put together a scrapbook. (For more background on Romeo see Introduction and Joaquin, this volume). Instead of the warm interaction I was hoping for, I found the experience to be not only affectively flat, but even alienating (Mates, 28 November, 2006: fieldnotes). About a picture with people not previously presented, he said only, *This is Warren and Carrie,*[1] without further explanation. Later commenting on another photograph he explained too much saying, *This is my wife Juliet.* This particular instance really struck me as strange and inappropriate because she was not a stranger to me. Juliet had introduced us to one another; she was in another room of the house at the time; she suggested we make the scrapbook. Did Romeo think I was a stranger that needed this kind of explanation? I left that day wondering what about our interaction was so off-putting and whether frontal lobe degeneration could predict this change in interactional capacity. In this chapter, I will first review how normals (people without neurological deficits) organize their third-person, person reference formulations (PRFs) when talking about photographs. Then I will present both the ways in which FTD patients conform

---

1.　All names have been changed, but the utterances otherwise remain the same in form.

to and depart from those norms. Finally, the problems these FTD patients present with in their PRFs will be used to build a potential neurobiological account for third-person, person reference in interaction.

**Person Reference Formulations in Normals in a Photograph Narrative Activity**

When we examine the structure of ordinary conversation, we can observe the many ways in which *recipient design* is an organizing principle. This phenomenon refers to displays in the talk by which the speaker gives a nod to the knowledge or point of view of the recipient or interlocutor (Sacks *et al.* 1974). In their seminal work on PRF in conversation, Sacks and Schegloff (1979) elucidated two organizing principles, the first of which stems from the general principle of recipient design. The first principle being that, when possible, speakers design their formulations for their interlocutors by deploying *recognitional* forms that project the speaker's understanding of how the hearer knows the person being referred to. For example, a student may discuss the merits of *Mr. Smith* and not *my third period teacher* assuming that *Mr. Smith* sufficiently locates who the teacher is in the shared understanding between the student and his/her interlocutor. The second principle is that in achieving recognition, speakers tend to use the most minimal form available. *John,* in an utterance such as *John lit a bonfire in his backyard,* would be a minimal, recognitional PRF. *John* is recognitional because it specifies one particular John out of the many in the world based on shared knowledge and context between the speaker and hearer. The speaker can wrongly assume that *John* is a sufficient PRF for his/her recipient in which case either party can initiate fixing the problem. *John* is also minimal in that a descriptor such as *that neighbor of ours* (who is John) could also have been used as a recognitional, but it would not have been minimal. For a two-by-two matrix of PRFs see Table 1.

Because using recognitional PRFs relies on an assumption of shared knowledge, we might expect that they are used carefully so as not to be used in error. And indeed, in a study where ten individuals with no known neurological deficits reviewed 10-20 self-selected family photographs with a friend or acquaintance, these "normals" (in comparison with FTD patients) were very careful about using recognitionals when introducing someone for the first

|  | Recognitional | Non-recognitional |
|---|---|---|
| Minimal | *John* | *someone* |
| Non-Minimal | *that neighbor of ours* | *my uncle John* |

Table 1.    Example minimal/non-minimal, recognitional/non-recognitional person reference formulations

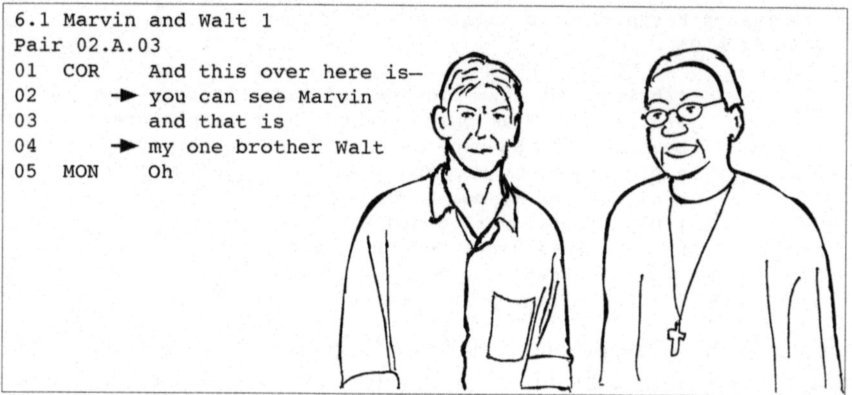


time in a set of photographs (Mates 2009). Interestingly, speakers were sensitive to both assuming too much and too little. The use of bare first names like *John* in the example was relatively rare (28 times out of 171 introductions, 16%) and tended to be reserved for immediate family members: children, spouses, and sometimes siblings.

### *Person reference formulations upon first appearance*

In example 6.1, Cora shows Mona a photograph of her husband and brother for the first time. They appear again in a subsequent photo and we will examine that sequence below.

Cora uses the bare first name *Marvin* (line 2) to identify her husband to her friend Mona, who knows that Cora is married to Marvin. In contrast, she uses a non-minimal, non-recognitional PRF *my one brother Walt* (line 4) which provides Mona with information about where Walt is situated in her social world. Mona's *oh* in line 5 signals her "change of state," meaning she shifted from not knowing to knowing something about Walt (Heritage 1984) and also signals her receipt of that information. Whether or not Mona actually knows to whom *Marvin* is referring, her response in the interaction does not make her knowledge of him or lack thereof relevant to the progress of the interaction. So we can say that the *oh* does not signal the deployment of the recognitional *Marvin* as being problematic even though we cannot know for sure that it is in fact not problematic.

In example 6.2, Jen identifies the women standing in the photograph in lines 8–9. For two of the women, she uses bare first names without any supplementary information about who they are to her, *That's Karen. That's Callie.* These women are her sisters and her deployment of those bare, first names relies on her belief that her hearer Penny knows her sisters by name independently and prior to this interaction. These classes of people, close family members, tend to be ones whose names might be shared because the names

```
6.2 That's Karen. That's Callie.
Pair 04.A.05

01   JEN     ((brings out next picture and turns it face down))
02           s(h)o(h) um I am only showing you this picture
03           because it's an own- because I had to show you
04           a picture of my mom and now that I realize I found
05           a picture of my mom I don't have to show this
06           ((flips photo over toward Patty))
07           which- m(h)a(h)n I look like a turtle. hh.
08       ➔   Okay, so that's my mom. (1.0) That's Karen. (1.4)
09       ➔   That's Callie. That's me.
```

uniquely identify people and thus facilitate reference to people who might be more frequently referred to. One also suspects that hearers might be held accountable to remember the names of such relations as a proxy for their investment in their relationship with the speaker.

This particular activity of reviewing photographs makes relevant two kinds of knowledge about third persons. Mona may know that Cora has a husband named Marvin, but may not know what he looks like if she had not met him in person before or seen him in a photograph. Speakers demonstrate a sensitivity to both of these categories of knowledge about a person as we see below.

In Example 6.3, Mona presents a photo and overtly comments on the knowledge she believes Cora to have with *and you know Marina* (line 2) to which Cora responds with an enthusiastically stretched *Ye:s* (line 3). The *you know* overtly claims knowledge about Cora's ability to visually identify Marina and in concordance with that claim of knowledge, the PRF is a bare, first name recognitional, *Marina*. This phenomenon is similarly displayed in Example 6.4. Here, Jen first identifies her daughters with recognitional PRFs using bare first names, *So this is Portia and Celeste* and immediately follows with *which you know* (line 2).

In examples 6.3 and 6.4, the *you know*s plus recognitional PRFs mark these

```
6.3 You know Marina
Pair 02.B.13

01   MON     ((Clicking to open photo on computer))
02   MON ➔   Ts and you know Marina
03   COR     Ye:s. Oh cute


6.4 Portia and Celeste which you know
Pair 04.A.01

01   JEN     ((pulls out photo))
02       ➔   So this is Portia and Celeste which you know.
03   PNN     Mm hmm:
```

people as known in their social relationship to the speaker and suggests that they are also known in their likeness. The speakers are pointing out that they are not telling their interlocutors anything new on either dimension.

Many study participants selected photos that included extended family members and friends. In fact, these make up the bulk of the people represented in the photographs. While these relatives and friends were near and dear to the speakers, their interlocutors did not know who these people were and how they were significant. For these interlocutors, speakers rarely used recognitional PRFs, except those speakers who had particularly close relationships with their interlocutors. For previously unfamiliar people, the speakers' first order of business was to situate the person in the speaker's social world. This took the form of many relational terms: *my mom, my dad, my cousin, my aunt, my son, my brother-in-law, one of my closest friends, a random woman we met that day, my high school sweetheart*. A full 80% of the introductions (137/171) began by describing the relationship of the referent to the speaker. Mothers and fathers were never additionally identified by name in the data collected. Of the 137 introductions that situated the person in the speaker's social world, 57 were additionally identified by name (42%). Only on five occasions out of 171 introductions (3%) did a speaker first name a person and then subsequently situate them in his/her social world.

In example 6.5, Sarah in lines 3-4 identifies three boys in a photo from the 1950s. Two of them are her older brothers whom she has previously identified and introduced to the recipient, Carla. She names them using bare, first-name recognitionals, *Larry* and *Bill*. Continuing in that vein of bare, first-name recognitionals, she identifies the third boy as *Doug*, pauses and then locates him in her social world as her uncle. The pause suggests that Sarah became aware after her deployment of the recognitional that it might not have been sufficient and adds *my uncle* to fix the potential problem. This fix points again to another organizing principle in PRF in a photograph narrative activity, that speakers prioritize the nature of the social relationship over the name identity of a person. The nature of the relationship between a speaker and the person in his/her photographs is more important than their name so sometimes only the relationship is given, and when the name is given, it tends to be placed after the relational term or description.

Whether or not someone is named before or after being located in the

```
6.5 Doug my uncle
Pair 06.A.12


01   CAR     ((Pointing))
02           This looks like it come- could come from Our Gang
03   SAR     Yea and that's um Larry, (0.6) And I think that's Bill,
04      ➜    and that must be Doug (.) my uncle.
```

speaker's social world may have interactional implications if that person shows up in a later photograph. Often people appeared more than once in a set of photographs. Unless the person showed up in back to back photos and looked physically similar in those photos, speakers usually treated the 2nd through Nth appearance of a person as part of a new interactional sequence and referred to them with a full noun phrase instead of a pronoun. Even if the photos were sequential, if there was a potential for mis-identification because of a significant age difference of a person between photographs or if a face was partially obscured, then there was a tendency to re-identify the person without reintroducing the relationship of the person to the speaker.

### Person reference formulations on 2nd to Nth appearances

If we return to Example 6.1, we see Marvin and Walt introduced for the first time. In the photograph, they are in the foreground, easy to see and both facing the camera. In the next photograph, seen below in Example 6.6, Walt is in profile in the foreground and wearing sunglasses which he did not have on in the previous photograph. Marvin is in the middle ground facing the camera wearing a different kind of sunglasses and his body is partially obscured by a little girl.

When Cora shows this photograph, she begins by locating the setting, the castle in the background (not in transcript). Then she names the people in the photograph. She starts in the foreground in the bottom right of the photograph with *and that's Walt again* (line 1). The use of *Walt* as a recognitional is appropriate because his place in her social world was established in the description of the previous photo with *my one brother Walt*. Following his name is *again* which indexes her use of *Walt* not as an introduction for the first time but a re-identification. *Walt* as Cora's brother was already established, but it could be difficult to tell that this particular person in the photograph is him. In line 3, Cora identifies the little girl and finally she identifies the last person in the photo with *and that's young Marvin* (line 5). Marvin is her husband and

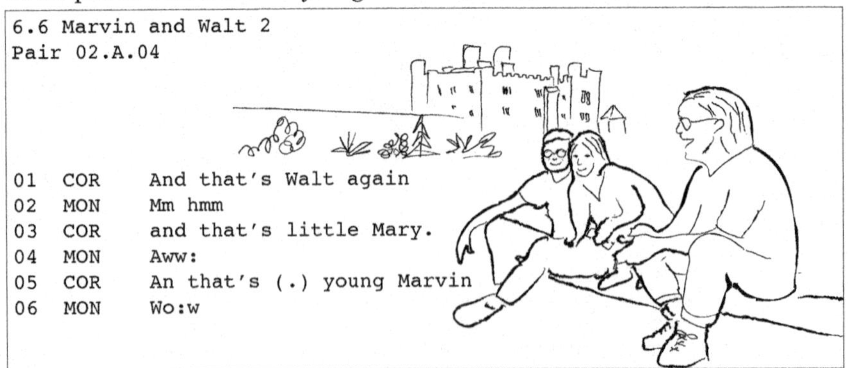

was introduced in the previous photo with the bare, first-name recognitional form, as discussed earlier. Here the modifier *young* provides the account for the re-identification. It shows that there is a time difference between the two photos in addition to Marvin being visually more difficult to recognize. Cora avoids the problem of mis-identification here again and gives an account of the possible trouble source as motivation for her re-identification of Marvin.

To summarize the features of person reference in normals in a photograph narrative activity, we can say:

1. Bare, first-name recognitionals are used sparingly for initial reference but when possible.

2. People who cannot be referred to with recognitionals are overwhelmingly introduced by their location in the speaker's social world, which takes priority over providing a name

3. In 2nd to Nth mentions, speakers are sensitive to "previous-ness" and the possibility of mis-identification.

### Person Reference in Frontotemporal Dementia in a Photographic Narrative Activity

In the next section, I will document some of the features of FTD PRF in a similar photograph narrative activity comparing their performance with the patterns described previously. The section will only compare and contrast without attempting to explain why any departures might have occurred.

### *Case 1: Romeo*

The first subject to be examined is Romeo, who was described in the introduction and in Joaquin's chapter. Unlike the participants in the other study who were asked to review photos with an acquaintance as part of a research study, Romeo and the researcher (Andrea Mates) reviewed photographs together in the course of a longer participant-observation ethnography. On this day, Romeo's wife Juliet asked them to review a large stack of photos from the previous year and to select those that documented his confirmation into the Catholic Church, which had taken place a few months prior. This makes the activity different from the studies reviewed in the previous section because Romeo was not being asked to simply review photos with Andrea but to review them as a step toward accomplishing something else. Together they were asked to select a subset of the photos for a scrapbook commemorating a particular event. Nevertheless, we can see in the interaction that Romeo encounters the same issues that normals face; namely how to refer to someone in their first appearance in a set of photos and then how to make reference to them in subsequent photos.

**First appearance person reference formulations**

Looking at the first photo at the top of the pile, Romeo starts off well. Andrea begins the sequence by asking *So who are these people* (line 2). This utterance requests information which Andrea may or may not already have. In this instance, in fact, she does not know who these people are. Romeo responds with *Tha- that's uh my family at home* (line 3–4). The reference to the people collectively as *my family* is appropriately non-recognitional and also situates them in a particular domain of his social world as his kin. In line 7, Andrea asks for greater specificity, asking *who's who?* Pointing to each one in turn, Romeo starts with the right most person and says, *That- that's meh dad* (line 8). This formulation [this/that is] + [parent reference] was how normals usually first introduced their parents (Only one person introduced his parents as *Dad. Mom.* without the [this/that is] in front). Romeo's PRF locates the precise social relationship of the person to the speaker and does so uniquely since all humans have one biological father. The form does not suppose any *a priori* knowledge about his father on the part of the hearer.

After Andrea's acknowledgement token in line 9, Romeo continues with an introduction to the person seated next to his father. He begins his utterance (line 10) with *That's my s-* but cuts himself off and reformulates his utterance as *that's our sister Pam. My sister Pam* would have utterly coincided with the pattern of non-recognitional PRF used by the normals. However, the reformulated version *Our sister Pam* is problematic because it is unclear who belongs in the pronoun *our. The our* presumes some knowledge that Andrea does not have. Having created one locus of trouble, Romeo moves on to deploy a PRF that differs from the patterns of normals, *and that is Sally* (line 10). The circle of people that interlocutors referred to using recognitionals was very small—usually limited to spouses and children

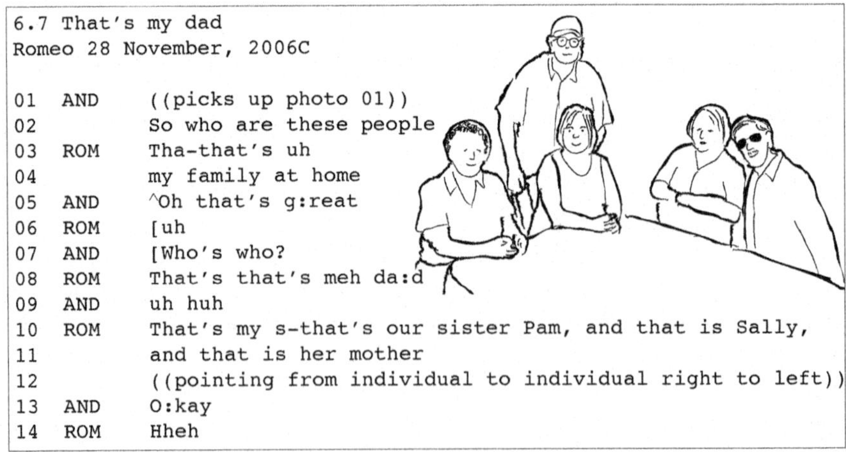

```
6.7 That's my dad
Romeo 28 November, 2006C

01   AND      ((picks up photo 01))
02            So who are these people
03   ROM      Tha-that's uh
04            my family at home
05   AND      ^Oh that's g:reat
06   ROM      [uh
07   AND      [Who's who?
08   ROM      That's that's meh da:d
09   AND      uh huh
10   ROM      That's my s-that's our sister Pam, and that is Sally,
11            and that is her mother
12            ((pointing from individual to individual right to left))
13   AND      O:kay
14   ROM      Hheh
```

and in the case of pairs acquainted through work, co-workers. Siblings were only referred to with recognitional PRFs between pairs that were particularly well acquainted. It turns out that Sally is Juliet's younger sister and Romeo's sister-in-law. Using a bare, first name as a recognitional is inappropriate here because the relational status of Sally and her very existence had never been mentioned previously. There was no opportunity for Andrea too know *a priori* who Sally was. The patterns of interaction between normals suggests that any of the following *non*-recognitional PRFs would have been more appropriate: *my wife's sister* or *my sister-in-law*. Telling Andrea this woman's name is *Sally* should have been Romeo's secondary concern that came after establishing her relationship with him.

The final introduction, *that is her mother* (line 11), is appropriate in this context. While in fact this woman is his mother-in-law and *this is my mother-in-law* would be the more proximal relationship term, he has not located Sally in his social world as a relation of his and this woman is indeed Sally's mother. This *her* refers back to Sally, the immediately preceding female referent, and *mother* uniquely locates the woman in Sally's social world. What we observe then is that Romeo has a range of competence in his first mentions. *That's my dad* and *that's her mother* are formulated appropriately as expected from the study on normals. *Our sister Pam* is not trouble free, but it does not treat this person as someone that the hearer should be able to locate independently. *That is Sally*, on the other hand, makes an incorrect claim about the prior knowledge of the hearer. It presumes that Sally's relationship to the speaker is already known when it is not.

## 2nd to Nth appearance person reference formulations

In addition to problems with his formulations for first appearances. Romeo displays problems in his formulations for 2nd to Nth appearances as well. In the second photo in the set, Example 6.8, Romeo picks up the photo and suggests that unlike the first photo perhaps this second one might be appropriate for his scrapbook. Andrea responds to the suggestion by asking *Who are these people* (line 5). In this context the question can operate as a request for both an introduction to the persons in the photo as well as an account for why these people would belong in the scrapbook. Romeo's telling is insufficient on both counts.

In lines 6–8, Romeo slowly lists the three people seated at the table: Warren, Carrie, and Juliet's mother. *Warren* and *Carrie* appear for the first time, and in this position the PRFs used are usually sensitive to either locating the referent in the speaker's social world or signaling a belief about the recipient's knowledge of the referent's relationship to the speaker through the use of a recognitional. *Warren* and *Carrie* are formulated to fall into the later category

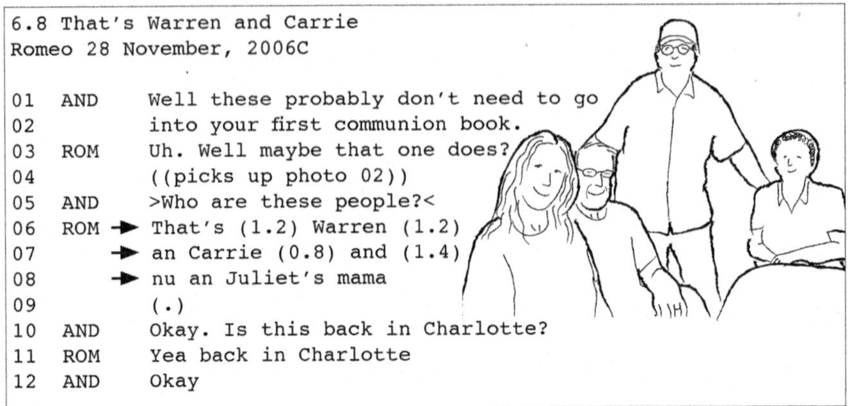

```
6.8 That's Warren and Carrie
Romeo 28 November, 2006C

01  AND      Well these probably don't need to go
02           into your first communion book.
03  ROM      Uh. Well maybe that one does?
04           ((picks up photo 02))
05  AND      >Who are these people?<
06  ROM  ➤   That's (1.2) Warren (1.2)
07       ➤   an Carrie (0.8) and (1.4)
08       ➤   nu an Juliet's mama
09           (.)
10  AND      Okay. Is this back in Charlotte?
11  ROM      Yea back in Charlotte
12  AND      Okay
```

(lines 6–7) but do so inappropriately because these people are unknown to Andrea. She has no prior knowledge about them and does not even know that they exist. *Juliet's mama* is a non-recognitional and does locate her in his social world as his wife's mother. In this sense, the formulation is appropriate. It is not without trouble because the same woman in the same room but at a different angle was previously referred to as Sally's mother (Example 6.7, line 11). We will not dwell on this because our concern here is how *Warren* and *Carrie* will be referred to the next time they appear in the set, which is five photographs later in the seventh photograph.

In the second appearance of Warren and Carrie in Example 6.9, Romeo begins with *That's Carrie* after Romeo seems to have aborted his attempt to talk about the photograph and is prompted by Andrea to identify the people in the photograph (lines 1–6). Romeo begins in the same manner as before, using a recognitional PRF, the bare first-name *That's Carrie* (line 7). But he reformulates this by repeating his utterance and replacing her name with a non-recognitional *That's my sister* (line 8). The non-recognitional establishes her place in his social world, which he had not done previously.

As a first mention, this formulation of name followed by social relationship is more rare than the social relationship followed by a name, but it is not un-heard of as was shown above in Example 6.5. However, as a formulation for a second or otherwise subsequent appearance, this recognitional formulation to *non*-recognitional *re*-formulation is nowhere to be found in the normals data. For normals, the nature of their first appearance formulation informs subsequent mentions. If they introduce someone by social relationship only, then they continue with that reference. *My son* with no name will be *my son* in subsequent appearances. *My brother John* gives both the social relationship of the person and a name that uniquely identifies him. When speakers have thus introduced someone, on subsequent appearances, they usually forego

```
6.9 That's Carrie...my sister
Romeo 28 November, 2006C

01   AND      ((Picking up photo 07))
02   ROM      N then that's
03            (2.1)
04   AND      ((holding photo in ROM's
05            direction))
06            Who is this?
07   ROM  ➤  That's Carrie
08        ➤  that's my sister
09        ➤  and that's Warren
10            (.)
11   AND      You all have the same name
12   ROM      Yea. yea we do
13   AND      hih heh heh
```

the social relevance description and use the bare name (Mates 2009). Much less troubled is Romeo's next reference, which is to Warren. Here in line 9, his PRF is identical to his previous PRF in Example 6.8 *That's Warren*. The PRF is less troubled in that it consistently references the person Warren with a recognitional. It is potentially troubled in that there is a tendency for normals to index people who appear in such situations (i.e. more than once without the possibility of mis-identification) as having been mentioned previously. So if we forgive the inappropriate use of the recognitional in Example 6.8, in this instance, we could expect *That's Warren* + *again*.

### Case 2: Juno

Another subject in the FTD ethnography project was "Juno" a 62 year old, single, Caucasian woman. She had an adult daughter who lived elsewhere in the same city. She lived alone in her house but had two full-time caregivers; one lived with her during the week and another came on weekends. While also having a diagnosis of FTD, her behavioral manifestations were different from Romeo's primarily in that she initiated more of her own activities and verbalizations. Previously, she had bouts of aggressive behavior and was prescribed seroquel to moderate those behaviors. Like Romeo, she had spent time as an adult school educator but had also been a private investigator. She was a Peace Corps volunteer to Africa in the sixties and was a long time local activist.

Because she had a history of heavy drinking, alcohol-related frontal atrophy was a possible diagnosis early on, but the neurologist later changed the diagnosis to FTD and maintained the diagnosis after re-examination. Magnetic resonance imaging five years prior to the visit date from which the extracts below are drawn showed nothing remarkable about her ventricles, unlike Romeo, but there was some suggestion of microvascular atrophy in her frontal horns (Mates, 19 March, 2007: fieldnotes).

I (A. Mates) first visited Juno with L. Mikesell at her home in November of 2006. Upon first arrival, she kept asking what we were doing and if we were done yet, which was rather unsettling and unwelcoming. This turned out to be a feeling we usually had when spending time with her either at her home or her adult day care center. During a walk in a nearby park later that visit, she was more pleasant, making a point to ask our names and telling us stories.

The past seemed to provide her with a comfortable set of stories and opinions to share. This past included decades-old stories from her Peace Corps days to her civil rights activist days on up to very recent past experiences. She had gone with a friend to see a controversial movie, *Borat,* the day before and expressed disgust and offense at the movie content. She often listened to progressive talk radio and commented on recent news events with us. Around the time of our visit, there had been a controversial taser incident at our university, and when she found out that we were affiliated with this university, she made a point to comment on the incident. While Juno had much to say about the past, future events and plans were difficult to project. We asked her what she would do later that day after we left, and she said she would work on her book about her time in Africa. Her daughter was visibly surprised at this utterance and later assured us that it was unlikely Juno would actually be doing that.

Seventeen months later, L. Mikesell and I brought along two other ethnographers on a visit with her to see if their fresh perspective would offer us new insights into her social practices. During that visit to her home, because the new ethnographers had never been there before, we asked her to show us around and to tell us about the many family photographs she had on the walls. In her tellings about her family photographs, she initiated the introductions without prompting and sometimes gave accompanying stories. This differs from Romeo's general lack of proactive engagement in the activity. However, Juno still exhibited some problems with both her introductions to people in their first appearance as well as her re-references to them in their second through Nth appearances.

### First appearance person reference formulations

In Example 6.10, we see the many ways in which Juno succeeds in deploying appropriate PRFs. In this excerpt, she is pointing to a set of framed photographs on one wall in a stairway which had photos on both walls. Going from frame to frame she narrates what is going on or who is represented in the photographs.

In line 6, *This is my mom* is not her mom's first appearance in the activity.

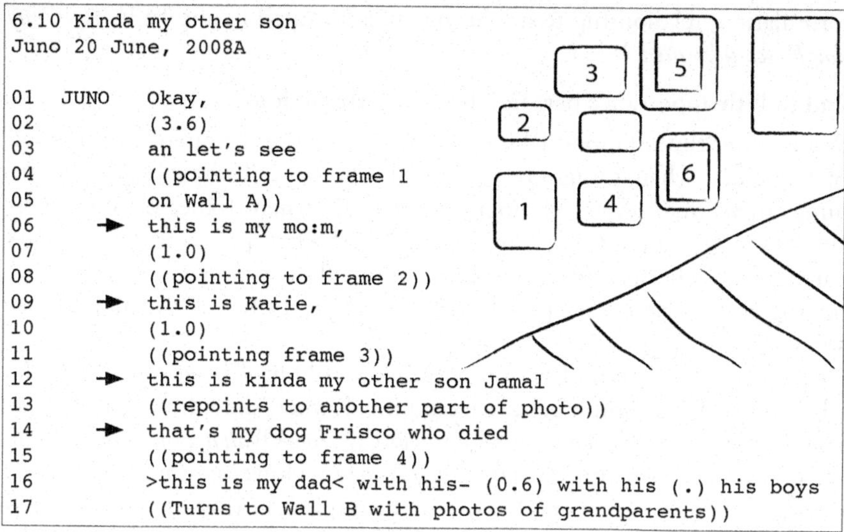



```
6.10 Kinda my other son
Juno 20 June, 2008A

01   JUNO      Okay,
02             (3.6)
03             an let's see
04             ((pointing to frame 1
05             on Wall A))
06      ➙      this is my mo:m,
07             (1.0)
08             ((pointing to frame 2))
09      ➙      this is Katie,
10             (1.0)
11             ((pointing frame 3))
12      ➙      this is kinda my other son Jamal
13             ((repoints to another part of photo))
14      ➙      that's my dog Frisco who died
15             ((pointing to frame 4))
16             >this is my dad< with his- (0.6) with his (.) his boys
17             ((Turns to Wall B with photos of grandparents))
```

There were a number of photos with her mother in them downstairs where the group had been previously reviewing family photographs. However, the photos around the house captured her mother at different ages with different styles of photography, so Juno's re-referencing could be construed as avoiding mis-identification and might not be expected to index previous-ness in the way that Romeo's re-referencing of Warren was in Example 6.9. In line 9, *This is Katie* is an introduction to someone who has not been referenced previously. There was a framed photograph of Katie on the mantle downstairs, but it had been skipped over in the narration. So in terms of the interaction, this is Katie's first appearance that is being made relevant to the activity. The use of the bare first-name marks it as a recognitional in which Juno is claiming that her hearers already know Katie's relationship to her, and this is indeed the case. Katie is Juno's daughter and has durable power of attorney over her mother's affairs. The researchers had been working with Katie over the course of the study to arrange visits with Juno. This is an example of a canonical use of a recognitional to introduce someone over the course of a photograph narrative activity. Finally, in line 12, Juno gives a standard introduction for a previously unknown third person using a non-recognitional PRF; *This is kinda my other son Jamal.* The formulation begins by locating the person in her social world and then provides the uniquely identifying first name. While the relationship is not a straightforwardly biological one as shown by *kinda,* and *my other son* contrasts the relationship with the implied daughter relationship she has with Katie, the information supplied does place him in close proximity to her and explains why a young African-American teenager warrants a framed photograph in her stairwell of family photographs. This formulation, relationship term plus name, is repeated in line 14 in *That's my dog Frisco who died.*

### 2nd to Nth appearance person reference formulations

While often times Juno's PRFs were unproblematic, she rarely ever indexed previous-ness when it might be warranted. On the wall where Jamal's picture hung, there were several photographs of Katie where Katie was unmistakably Katie (Example 6.11, lines 4 and 12). Unlike photographs of Juno's parents where her parents might be in group shots from decades ago, these photographs of Katie were posed portraits of Katie by herself and all from her adolescence.

The expected pattern of person reference would have been something like what Cora did in Example 6.1 and Example 6.6, where she either acknowledges that the person has been mentioned previously, *That's Walt again,* or gives some account for the re-naming, *That's young Marvin.* However, Juno does not do this in either re-mention of Katie here in Example 6.11 (lines 4 and 12, *This is Katie*) or in the many instances where Katie or her parents appear unmistakably identifiable in other photographs. In fact, Juno is so out of sync with previous-ness that she redecribes photo frame 3 (Example 6.11, line 4) even though she had already done so two to three minutes earlier in Example 6.10, line 12 (*This is kinda my other son Jamal*).

The staccato identification of Katie and her parents over and over again without anything signaling that she recognized that they had been previously mentioned gave the interaction a rote, test-like quality as if her task was to name the people rather than to share something about her life and loved ones with interested co-participants. This feeling on my part persisted despite the anecdotes about various people that she occasionally sprinkled in.

In this section, we have documented trouble in FTD PRFs without trying to explain why FTD brain degeneration might lead to such troubles. In

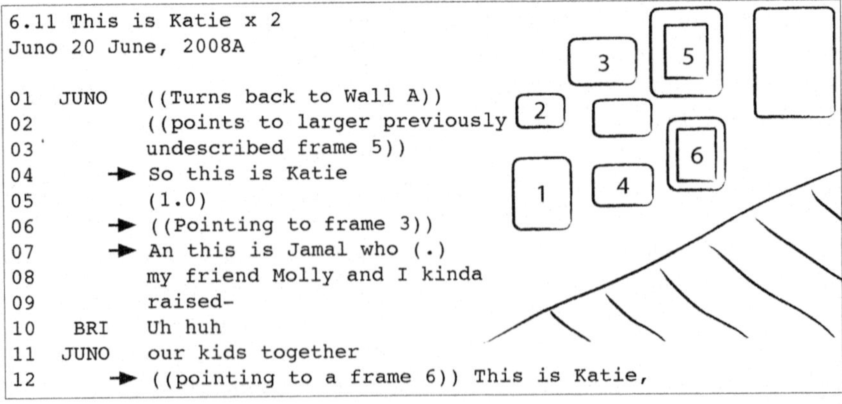

```
6.11 This is Katie x 2
Juno 20 June, 2008A


01    JUNO    ((Turns back to Wall A))
02            ((points to larger previously
03            undescribed frame 5))
04        ➤   So this is Katie
05            (1.0)
06        ➤   ((Pointing to frame 3))
07        ➤   An this is Jamal who (.)
08            my friend Molly and I kinda
09            raised-
10    BRI     Uh huh
11    JUNO    our kids together
12        ➤   ((pointing to a frame 6)) This is Katie,
```

the next section, we will explore this question by first considering what the nature of the troubles are and then what cognitive processes may be disrupted by FTD brain degeneration.

## A Case for the Problems in Ftd Person Reference Formulations

Unlike the normals in their photograph naming activity, these two FTD patients' interactions lack the precision tracking and attention to their interlocutors' knowledge sets from moment to moment. This was manifested in a number of different ways. Romeo's use of recognitional PRFs for *Warren and Carrie* over-supposes and under-tells. While Schegloff (2007) examines self-references and ordinary phone conversations to show that interlocutors over-suppose and under-tell as a "social-affiliational imperative (Enfield *et al.* 2007)" so as to credit the hearer with more knowledge rather than less, there was no warrant for such credit here. Romeo's *That is Carrie. That is my sister* and Juno's repeated *This is Katie* fails to mark the subsequent appearances as subsequent and thus fails to mark that they are doing something different from a first mention about a first appearance.

Romeo's *my wife Juliet*, which was mentioned in the beginning of the chapter, was so marked it spurred two years of investigation. *My wife Juliet* has the opposite properties of *Warren and Carrie* in that it under-supposes and over-tells. Over-telling is interactionally sanctionable (Heritage 2007; Schegloff 2007) as we can see below in Example 6.12 where Cora points out her pet as *the doggie* (line 5) instead of using a recognitional PRF. Mona responds by giving the dog's name, *Minty* (line 6), which demonstrates her knowledge and pushes back on Cora's formulation which suggests that Mona would not know who Minty was if simply referred to by his name.

This instability in FTD PRF, variously over- and under-telling, could result from the inability to infer the knowledge states of others or from the lack of motivation to do the inferring or a combination of the two. If the ability is impaired, then the patients would be displaying deficits in theory of mind, also called perspective taking. If the ability is intact but not being applied, then perhaps there is a motivation deficiency that impinges on applying effort to sustaining social relationships.

```
 6.12 Oh: Minty
 Pair 02.A.6


 01   COR      So that's him and this is-
 02            (0.4)
 03   MON      Oh::
 04   COR      a rare family photo because um usually of course
 05         ➤ Mary isn't there.  And that's the doggie.
 06   MIN  ➤ Oh: Minty
```

### Impairments in theory of mind and perspective taking

Theory of mind, the ability to infer the knowledge or belief of another particularly in its potential difference from one's own, was first suggested as its own cognitive capacity by Premack and Woodruff (1978). In the intervening 30 years a great deal of energy has been spent on understanding what this phenomenon might be as a psychological, developmental, and neurobiological construct. There have been increasing concerns from scholars of interaction regarding the label *theory of mind* (Antaki 2004; Danziger 2006; Schegloff 2006) and some in the field have moved on to call the phenomenon *perspective taking* (Mason and Macrae, 2008). I will follow this convention.

Research has shown that children develop increasingly complex understandings of perspective taking as they mature. First order false belief is simply the understanding that I know that you believe something different from what I know; for instance, if I saw a ball moved while you were out of the room, I would think that you believed the ball was in its original location. This basic level of perspective taking is well developed by the time children are three to four years of age (Wimmer and Perner 1983). Second order false belief is the more complex understanding that I know that you think that I think X even though X is not the case; for example, if you are unaware that I was peeking through a window and saw you move the ball while I was out of the room, then I would expect that you believe that I think the ball is in its original location. Six-to-eight year olds begin to consistently perform well on this kind of a task (Stone *et al.* 1998). Late developing is the ability to identify faux pas, to be able to infer what another person may feel in a particular social context. Children do not begin performing consistently on these sorts of tasks until 11 years of age (Stone *et al.* 1998).

Mason and Macrae's (2008) review of perspective taking implicates the following neuroanatomical regions: the temporo-parietal junction, the superior temporal sulcus, and the medial prefrontal cortex (mPFC). FTD often begins with degeneration along a medial prefrontal-anterior temporal axis (Mendez, personal communication, 19 March, 2007). Thus with regard to the neurobiology involved in perspective taking, the temporo-parietal junction and superior temporal sulcus would be preserved, but the contribution of the ventral medial prefrontal cortex would likely begin weakening as the frontal lobe degeneration progresses. The mPFC has been highlighted in a number of studies that test more complex attributions of psychological states (Gallagher *et al.* 2002; Mitchell *et al.* 2005; Rilling *et al.* 2004). Shamay-Tsoory *et al.* (2005) reported that damage in this medial prefrontal region left subjects with the ability to infer beliefs about others but not feelings. This is consistent with reports that FTD patients can correctly handle first and second-order false belief tasks which test the ability to understand that others can have different beliefs from one's own. However, when asked to identify faux pas, which ask about the emotional state of another, FTD patients perform significantly worse than age-matched Alzheimer's patients (Gregory *et al.* 2002).

In selecting an interactionally appropriate person reference formulation out of a list of candidate PRFs, the ability to infer the beliefs or knowledge of another is critical particularly if there is reason to believe that one's interlocutor knows a third person only in a particular way or setting or does not know a person at all. However, is the ability to infer the *feelings* of another also critical? Given that FTD patients typically still have intact first- and second-order false belief, in order for perspective-taking impairment to explain their problems with deploying PRFs appropriately, one must establish a particular role for the inferring of feelings over beliefs or knowledge in the process.

It is helpful to consider appropriateness as falling along two dimensions: First, does the PRF sufficiently identify who is being referred to? As we saw in Example 6.5, where a bare, first-name recognitional *Doug* might be possibly insufficient, the speaker adds on a description of his relationship to herself, *my uncle,* after a hearable micro-pause. A second dimension of appropriateness asks whether the PRF indexes ones relationship to both the referent and one's interlocutor as one intends? One can intentionally accomplish more than simply referring by modifying the PRF. Stivers (2007) documents the use of alternative recognitionals as categorical shifts between possible recognitional forms that mark the reference as a social action doing more than referring to a person. In her central example, Nicole speaks with her mother about her mother's sister Alene, but instead of referring to Aunt Alene as *Aunt Alene* or *Alene,* Nicole formulates the reference as *yer s̲:ister*, pushing the association of this person away from herself toward her mother. Nicole does this in the larger context of formulating a complaint and her PRF subserves that objective. Nicole's complaint happens to be against both her mother and her aunt and the PRF *yer s̲:ister* handily both distances the aunt from Nicole and attaches the aunt to Nicole's mother.

In stark contrast, where FTD subjects depart from the expected PRF there is no interactional sense that they are intentionally trying to accomplish more than to simply refer to that particular person. In Example 6.7, Romeo's PRFs come in a list as he introduces a group of people. None of these people are known to Andrea so there are no alternative recognitional forms to choose from although there are certainly any number of descriptive non-recognitionals that could be used. When the bare, first-name recognitional *Sally* (line 11) is used, it is inappropriate both because it insufficiently identifies who she is in his social world and also because the PRF can be seen as making an assumption about the nature of Romeo's relationship with Andrea that is not true—that they are acquainted enough for Andrea to know his extended family. On the other hand, Romeo's *my wife Juliet* adequately situates her in his social world; however, it indexes a relationship so distant that Andrea would possibly not know that he is married and would not know that his wife's name is Juliet. Had the PRF been only *my wife* it might be seen as performing two functions: identifying someone difficult to make out in a photograph which normals did as necessary and highlighting the intimacy of their relationship and his tenderness toward her through the deployment of an alternative recognitional. *Juliet* would be the unmarked, doing-nothing-more-than-referring PRF. But together *my wife Juliet* takes on a completely non-recognitional form that indexes a social distance greater than what existed between the interlocutors.

Impaired abilities to infer the feelings of others while inferences about others' knowledge or belief remain intact may lead to a misevaluation of the consequences of deploying an inappropriate PRF. Assuming first some mental catalog of PRFs that would identify a particular person such as *my wife, Juliet, her, my wife Juliet,* the ability to infer the feelings of another might weight different PRFs differently; some as relationship maintaining, enhancing or detracting, and the valuation a particular PRF received would depend on the specific interlocutor. There is literature that suggests that social strain and isolation affects the anterior cingulate in a manner similar to physical pain (Eisenberger and Lieberman 2004). Just as people avoid physical pain, they have reason to avoid social isolation. Functioning abilities to infer the feelings of others should identify PRFs that might strain social relationships as formulations to be avoided. Just as speakers are sensitive to telling their interlocutors enough information suggesting that they want to avoid assuming too much knowledge on the part of their interlocutor, they are also sensitive to telling too much. So in Example 6.3, Mona carefully avoids suggesting that Cora might not be able to recognize Marina and thus avoids indexing a potential gap in their shared knowledge and lives. Her PRF *and you know Marina* (line 2) overtly asserts that Mona believes that Cora knows who Marina is and what Marina looks like and that between Mona and Cora exists the kind of relationship where that can be assumed. To have only introduced the person as *Marina* might have suggested that Mona is unsure whether Cora knows what Marina looks like causing trouble for their relationship (Heritage 2007, 277). In the FTD data, the patients' PRFs lack the this level of sensitivity, and when the PRFs are problematic with respect to ethnographic reports or as situated in the interaction, the FTD subjects themselves do not initiate a correction of the problems. Reports of impaired ability to infer the feelings of others in FTD may suggest that they are also unable to anticipate the relational consequences of a particular PRF leaving them with a type of relational blindness.

### *Impairments in social motivation*

A second possibility is that there is no relational blindness; first- and second-order false belief provide adequate cognitive support to select an interactionally appropriate PRF. Instead in FTD, medial prefrontal degeneration weakens social motivation and gives rise to a "Rhett Butler Effect" in which a person may be able to predict potential relational consequences, but does not care to ameliorate any deleterious effects.

Social motivation, as a psychological construct, posits a form of motivation toward relationship formation and maintenance which is more complex than motivations toward food, sex, and warmth for example. This is predicated on the evolutionary advantage of being part of a small interdependent group (Stevens and Fiske 1995) which developed into a fundamental drive to belong (Baumeister and Leary 1995).

As mentioned before, FTD is a focal type dementia; particular parts of the brain are affected but not all. The focus of the neurobiological account thus far has been the degeneration in the medial prefrontal cortex. Above we discussed the role of the medial prefrontal cortex (mPFC) in perspective taking, but here we are arguing that medial prefrontal degeneration may also affect the underlying neurobiology of affiliation, which we are arguing plays a critical role in social motivation.

Depue and Morrone-Strupinsky (2005) present a neurobiological model of affiliative bonding which implicates the ventral medial PFC (vmPFC) as the central component in forming an intensity-encoded incentive motivational state. (Their paper labels this region as the medial orbital cortex which we believe indexes the same region.) As they present it, the vmPFC assesses and plans engagement with the external world based on its predictions of the rewardingness of the action. It integrates discrete, explicit stimuli via reciprocal connection to the basolateral amygdala and to non-discrete, non-explicit stimuli via its reciprocal connection to the extended amygdala. These three regions, the vmPFC, basolateral amydala, and extended amygdala, massively innervate both the ventral tegmental area (VTA) and the nucleus accumbens shell (NAS). Based on the strength of input from these regions and the hippocampus which provides spatial and contextual information, the VTA releases dopamine (DA) which produces feelings of reward during the process of pursuing a goal. The contextual information from those four corticolimbic regions: the vmPFC, basolateral amygdala, extended amygdala and hippocampus, converges with the VTA DA projections on the dendrites of medium spiny neurons in the NAS. With enough activation from the corticolimbic projections and the VTA DA projections, long lasting, long term potentiation of these connections can be facilitated. This long term potentiation creates memories for rewards such as affiliative rewards and the contexts in which they occur (see Lee *et al.* 2009 for an application of this model to language acquisition).

In the neurobiology Depue and Morrone-Strupinski (2005) describe, because the vmPFC receives a constantly updated report on the degree of rewardingness of a situation via a pathway from the NAS through the ventral pallidum and dorsomedial thalamus, it is not just one player among many in these systems for reward and memories for rewards. It is an important node in a network for assessing and planning engagement with the external world.

With vmPFC degeneration, FTD patients may not receive enough reward signals to keep them on the path toward maintaining social relationships. To further compound the social problems that may be engendered by vmPFC degeneration, the vmPFC receives input from the fusiform gyrus and the superior temporal sulcus which process faces and biological motion. This would likely make more difficult processing other's interactional moves and the rewarding (or not rewarding) nature of a particular social engagement.

The claim here is not that FTD patients exhibit *no* goal seeking behaviors. The participant observation ethnography revealed particularly strong food seeking drives, for example. If food was visibly available, there was a tendency for the patients to move toward it. But acquiring food is different from building or even maintaining a social relationship. Food and hunger correspond with basic physiological changes in the body as blood sugar drops, taste buds encounter different food molecules, or the stomach expands over the course of a meal. Social relationships require the processing of more complex cues and the ability to maintain long-term, abstract goals. Memories about food experiences should still be available to FTD patients, acquiring food in a familiar environment should be possible, and they should still experience consummatory reward from eating. Rather the claim being proposed here is that *social* drives may be impaired as the vmPFC degenerates. That degeneration may be making it more difficult for FTD patients to integrate all the stimuli that would normally push them along a path toward socially appropriate, relationship maintaining behaviors. Thus, a second possible reason for FTD problems in PRF could be damage to this system such that they could know how a particular PRF might impact their relationship, but there is not enough vmPFC activation to move them to effortfully choose a particular PRF that will sustain rather than strain the relationship.

### *Impaired perspective taking and social motivation in feedback loops*

A final possibility is that these two systems described above interact with one another and both are necessary. Appropriate PRF may depend on some threshold level of both being able to infer how someone might feel about a particular formulation in a given context as well as having the motivation to make a choice that would best suit one's goals for the relationship with one's interlocutor. Diminished mPFC activation in the perspective taking system may result in inconsistent recognition that a particular PRF would add relational strain unintentionally. Without that recognition, the also diminished social motivational system does not apply effort to alter the discourse to be context sensitive and also is less able to integrate and respond to any cues from the interlocutor once that PRF has been deployed.

This section has attempted to take the cases of inappropriate person reference from the previous section and examine some functions of regions degenerating in FTD in order to provide a potential neurobiological account for their verbal behavior. In fact, we do not know if any of the proposed neurocognitive processes accurately describe the brain-behavior link. However, the possibilities are being presented as hypotheses for further testing and to demonstrate one way in which a neurobiology of language can be built. In the next section this theory building process is taken one step further.

## A Neurobiology of Person Reference

In the previous section, the case was made that FTD impairments in perspective taking and/or social motivation was destabilizing their PRFs. If we examine the problematic PRFs, is there a remaining explanation for the PRFs that do get deployed, however inappropriately?

Returning to Example 6.8 in which Romeo identifies his brother-in-law and sister as *Warren* and *Carrie,* it appears that Romeo has chosen the reference forms that he himself has probably used most frequently. When he talks with his wife or other family members, *Warren* and *Carrie* are likely the forms that he uses. And he likely talks about them most often with people such as his wife who would know to whom these names refer. Unfortunately, his interlocutor in this instance was not familiar with them and Romeo's reference formulation does not take his interlocutor's perspective into account which gives his talk an air of misdirected egocentricity. This reliance on what he does most frequently is a reliance on procedural memory, a kind of implicit/nondeclarative memory (Schumann *et al.* 2004).

Procedural memory is encoded by repetitions of tasks or actions until they are automatized (Lee 2004). An example of proceduralized activity would be toothbrushing. Once the activity is initiated, the process is essentially on "auto-pilot." The toothbrusher gives little thought to his/her idiosyncratic toothbrushing motions. This becomes painfully apparent if the dentist recommends a new brushing technique. Initially, the new technique needs conscious guidance, but as it is repeated twice a day for a number of days, eventually this new technique will be proceduralized and toothbrushing can again go on "auto-pilot."

The neurobiology of procedural memory involves an early learning stage and an "overlearned" stage. These systems are described in detail in Lee (2004), but the pertinent details are that in the early learning stage the frontal lobe (presupplementary motor area) and the basal ganglia are recruited. But by the overlearned stage, primary activation is in subcortical regions, the cerebellar dentate nucleus and the posterior basal ganglia. Basal ganglia involvement is a careful balancing act between an excitatory "direct pathway" and an inhibitory "indirect pathway". Lee presents findings from research on language production on patients with Huntington's disease to link the basal ganglia and language use.

Procedural memory makes the most frequently used PRF out of a list of possibles the easiest to produce, requiring the least cognitive effort. However, the most used form will not always be the most appropriate form for the situation. In those situations, prefrontal inhibition of proceduralized subcortical pathways will be necessary in order for the uttered formulation to be recipient designed. For Romeo, when talking about his brother-in-law and sister, it's likely that *Warren* and *Carrie* are the proceduralized forms. And in most of his conversations about them, it is likely that the appropriate formulation and the proceduralized formulation are one and the same. But in this instance, they were not.

Because proceduralized memories are mostly encoded in the subcortical basal ganglia, they should be preserved in FTD patients. However, as we mentioned before, perspective taking abilities and social motivation degenerate with mPFC atrophy. FTD patients may be increasingly unable to use them to inhibit the proceduralized forms when needed.

While uninhibited proceduralized forms explain many of the inappropriate PRFs, this would not explain the highly marked *my wife Juliet*. One would imagine, and this is attested to by the ethnographic observations, that Romeo most frequently addressed his wife as *Juliet* and referred to her as *Juliet*. *My wife Juliet* appears neither appropriate nor resulting from the use of a proceduralized form. However, if we expand our scope of examination to the immediately preceding talk, we can hypothesize that this particular PRF may have been primed by the PRF *my cousin Bobby* (Example 6.13).

Perceptual priming is considered another form of implicit, non-declarative memory in which previous exposure to the same or similar stimuli will bias behavior in the response to a subsequent exposure to the stimulus (Henson 2003). In the selection of a particular person reference formulation out of a list of possible reference forms for a particular person, perceptual priming

```
6.13 My Wife Juliet
Romeo 28 November, 2006C

01   AND      >This looks like< somebody's backyard
02            (2.0)
03   ROM      Ahh (3.4) it is uh (5.3)
04        ➤  this is my (.) cousin Bobby
05   AND      mm-hmm
06            (0.7)
07   ROM   ➤ and this is my wife Juliet (0.8)
08            and uh I don't remember-I don't know
09            who all the rest of the people are=
10   AND      =Yea that's a lot of people
```

might weight the most recently used grammatical form more heavily than the other forms. In Example 6.13, it could be that the possessive + kin term + first name used in *my cousin Bobby* primed the same form used in *my wife Juliet*.

The neurobiology of priming is interesting in that much of it is expressed as regions of decreased hemodynamic activity. PET and fMRI measurements of brain activity during stage two report reductions in brain activity for both perceptual and conceptual priming. In tasks which attempt to isolate perceptual priming, the reduction is in posterior brain regions, in particular the extrastriate occipital cortex (Schacter and Buckner 1998). FTD patients typically do not have posterior degeneration, as such, it is likely that perceptual priming is a resource still available to them.

Table 2 summarizes the proposed neurobiology of person reference suggesting that person reference formulations are subject to the competition and cooperation of priming, procedural memory, perspective taking and social motivation which are each supported by largely different regions of the brain.

| Cognitive Bases of Person Reference | Neurobiology | Intact in FTD? |
|---|---|---|
| Perspective Taking | TPJ, STS | Yes |
|  | mPFC | NO |
| Social motivation | Amygdala, VTA, NAS | Yes |
|  | vmPFC | NO |
| Procedural memory | Basal Ganglia | Yes |
| Priming | Occipital cortex | Yes |

Table 2.    Neurobiology of person reference, VTA=Ventral Tegmental Area, NAS=Nucleus Accumbens, TPJ=Temporo-parietal Junction, STS=Superior Temporal Sulcus, (v)mPFC=(ventral) medial PFC.

FTD brain degeneration leaves most of the implicated regions untouched except for the mPFC which shows activation during tasks that involve inferring feelings and in higher order affiliative goal seeking behavior.

## Conclusion

The examination of FTD PRFs has accomplished much more than one could have anticipated initially. First, laying the participant-observation ethnography next to a conversation analytic documentation of breakdowns in FTD PRFs made clear how the PRFs play a role in the intricate building and sustaining of social relationships. This description is different but complementary to the work collected in *Person Reference in Interaction* (Enfield and Stivers 2007). Most noticeably, this work specifically examines the formulations of people with known neurocognitive deficits, and the problems in formulation are largely problems reported in the ethnographic field notes and not locally managed within the interaction. By methodological convention, the type of analysis in the Enfield and Stivers volume does not ask about the effect on the participants' relationship beyond what is manifested in the interaction itself. The ethnography here gave us a window into the relational effects of problems in PRF.

Second, because FTD brain degeneration is localized to the frontal lobes and temporal poles, this chapter was able to expand the efforts to understand frontal lobe contributions to language pragmatics. We were able to record and analyze the behavior of a population with reported social problems which would have been revealing in and of itself with regard to their deficits in language pragmatics (their language use in various social contexts). Additionally, we knew to a degree the way in which their brains were being particularly affected. While brain degeneration in FTD is unique in form and trajectory for each patient, by definition, FTD is not affecting the parietal and occipital cortex. Finally, all our subjects were screened to be predominantly right frontal atrophy FTD patients. And in this chapter, data from the subjects with temporal involvement were excluded. While there are a number of leaps being made in this chapter, the proposed neurobiology of person reference nevertheless has value. The neurobiological claims of this chapter are not to be taken as strong claims but rather as hypotheses for further exploration. The field of linguistics has long used language output to infer back to brain mechanisms. This chapter uses language output along with known functions of regions degenerating in FTD to develop theories about the brain-behavior link. It is unnecessary for the field to continue treating the brain as an unknowable black box.

Finally, this chapter has shown how participant observation ethnography in conjunction with conversation analysis can complement caregiver reports and cognitive tests for understanding populations with impaired social functions; not only those with FTD but also those suffering from autism, schizophrenia, post-traumatic stress disorder and some forms of traumatic brain injury. Caregivers have reported that FTD patients are egocentric and cognitive tests show deficiencies in affective perspective taking. The ethnography pointed to a particular locus of observation (PRFs) as being a potential source of social strain. Conversation analysis revealed ways in which their PRFs were missing the mark, particularly in that their PRFs did not adequately take their interlocutor's knowledge into account. Thus, when caregivers report that the patient is more egocentric, this global assessment may rest not just in a patient's single-minded pursuit of their own goals, but may also reflect caregivers' aggregate impressions of seemingly small but repeated infractions in conversational convention. When cognitive tests show deficiencies in inferring the feelings of others, what is the ecological validity of that test? This chapter presents one way of exploring the ecological validity of perspective taking tasks.

While this chapter accomplished more than initially anticipated, as often happens in the course of research, this line of inquiry has raised further questions. Now that it appears that PRF is a locus of investigation that may have both social science and clinical payoffs, could a diagnostic instrument be developed? A logical follow-up study would be to compare the rate of inappropriate PRFs with scores on perspective taking or social motivation measures. Are the relationships proposed here supported in an experimental setting? This could be done with not only FTD subject populations but also other populations with reported social deficits. How would we elicit PRFs? Is it possible to allow patients or subjects to self-select their own photographs and derive a meaningful clinical interpretation from their performance? For the neurobiology of language, can we better characterize or prove the roles of priming, procedural memory, perspective taking and social motivation in deploying appropriate PRF? Does this generalize to other pragmatic features in language use? There remains many questions unanswered and much work to be done.

## References

Antaki, C.

2004  Reading Minds or Dealing with Interactional Implications? *Theory & Psychology* 14(5): 667–683.

Baumeister, R.F. and M.R. Leary.

1995  The Need to Belong: Desire for Interpersonal Attachments as a Fundamental Human Motivation. *Pscyhological Bulletin* 117: 497–497.

Danziger, E.

2006 The thought that counts: Interactional consequences of variation in cultural theories of meaning. In *The Roots of Human Sociality,* edited by N.J. Enfield and S.C. Levinson, 259–278. Oxford: Berg.

Depue, R.A. and J.V. Morrone-Strupinsky.

2005 A neurobehavioral model of affiliative bonding: Implications for conceptualizing a human trait of affiliation. *Behavioral and Brain Sciences* 28(3): 313–350.

Eisenberger, N.I. and M.D. Lieberman.

2004 Why rejection hurts: a common neural alarm system for physical and social pain. *Trends in Cognitive Sciences* 8(7): 294–300.

Enfield, N.J., S. Kita and J.P. de Ruiter.

2007 Primary and secondary pragmatic functions of pointing gestures. *Journal of Pragmatics* 39(10): 1722–1741.

Enfield, N.J. and T. Stivers, eds.

2007 *Person Reference in Interaction.* Cambridge: Cambridge University Press.

Gallagher, H.L., A.I. Jack, A. Roepstorff and C.D. Frith.

2002 Imaging the intentional stance in a competitive game. *NeuroImage* 16(3,1): 814–821.

Gregory, C., S. Lough, V. Stone, S. Erzinclioglu, L. Martin, S. Baron-Choen, and J.R. Hodges.

2002 Theory of mind in patients with frontal variant frontotemporal dementia and Alzheimer's disease: theoretical and practical implications. *Brain* 125: 752–764.

Henson, R.N.A.

2003 Neuroimaging studies of priming. *Progress in Neurobiology* 70(1): 53–81.

Heritage, J.

1984 A Change of State Token and Aspects of Its Sequential Placement. In *Structures of Social Action,* edited by J.M. Atkinson and J. Heritage, 299–345. Cambridge: Cambridge University Press.

2007 Intersubjectivity and progressivity in person (and place) reference. In *Person Reference in Interaction: Linguistics, Cultural and Social Perspectives,* edited by N.J. Enfield and T. Stivers, 255–280. Cambridge: Cambridge University Press.

Lee, N.

2004 Neurobiology of procedural memory. In *The Neurobiology of Learning: Perspectives from Second Language Acquisition,* edited by J.H. Schumann, S.E. Crowell, N.E. Jones, N. Lee, S.A. Schuchert and L.A. Wood, 43–73. Mahwah, NJ: Lawrence Erlbaum Associates.

Lee, N., L. Mikesell, A.D.L. Joaquin, A.W. Mates and J. H. Schumann.

2009 *The Interactional Instinct: Language Evolution and Acquisition.* Oxford: Oxford University Press.

Mason, M.F., and C.N.Macrae.

2008 Perspective-Taking from a Social Neuroscience Standpoint. *Group Processes & Intergroup Relations* 11(2): 215–232.

Mates, A.W.

2009 What talking about them reveals about us: The organization of person reference in conversations about family photographs. Unpublished doctoral dissertation. University of California, Los Angeles.

Mitchell, J.P., M.R. Banaji and C.N. Macrae.

2005 The Link between Social Cognition and Self-referential Thought in the Medial Prefrontal Cortex. *Journal of Cognitive Neuroscience* 17(8): 1306–1315.

Premack, D. and G. Woodruff.

1978 Does the chimpanzee have theory of mind? *The Behavioral and Brain Sciences* 1(4): 515–526.

Rilling, J.K., A.G. Sanfey, J.A. Aronson, L.E. Nystrom and J.D. Cohen.

2004 The neural correlates of theory of mind within interpersonal interactions. *NeuroImage* 22: 1694–1703.

Sacks, H. and E.A. Schegloff.

1979 Two preferences in the organization of reference to persons in conversation and their interaction. *Everyday language: Studies in ethnomethodology*: 15–21.

Sacks, H., E.A. Schegloff and G. Jefferson.

1974 A simplest systematics for the organization of turn taking for conversation. *Language* 50: 696–735.

Schacter, D.L. and R. L. Buckner.

1998 Priming and the Brain. *NEURON-CAMBRIDGE MA-* 20: 185–195.

Schegloff, E.A.

2006 Interaction: The infrastructure for social institutions, the natural ecological niche for language, and the areana in which culture is enacted. In *The Roots of Human Sociality*, edited by N.J. Enfield and S.C. Levinson, 70–97. Oxford: Berg.

2007    Conveying who you are: the presentation of self, strictly speaking. In *Person Reference in Interaction: Linguistic, cultural and social perspectives*, edited by N.J. Enfield and T. Stivers, 123–148. Cambridge: Cambridge University Press.

Schumann, J.H., S.E. Crowell, N.E. Jones, N. Lee, S.A. Schuchert and L.A. Wood.

2004    *The Neurobiology of Learning: Perspectives from Second Language Acquisition.* Mahwah, NJ: Lawrence Erlbaum Associates.

Shamay-Tsoory, S.G., R. Tomer, B.D. Berger, D. Goldsher and J. Aharon-Peretz.

2005    Impaired affective theory of mind is associated with right ventromedial prefrontal damage. *Cog Behav Neurol* 18: 54–65.

Stevens, L.E. and S.T. Fiske.

1995    Motivation and cognition in social life: a social survival perspective. *Social cognition* 13(3): 189–214.

Stivers, T.

2007    Alternative recognitionals in person reference In *Person Reference in Interaction*, edited by N.J. Enfield and T. Stivers, 68–98. Cambridge: Cambridge University Press.

Stone, V.E., S. Baron-Cohen and R.T. Knight.

1998    Frontal lobe contributions to theory of mind. *Journal of Cognitive Neuroscience* 10(5): 640–656.

Wimmer, H. and J. Perner.

1983    Beliefs about beliefs: representation and constraining function of wrong beliefs in young children's understanding of deception. *Cognition* 13(1): 103–128.

— 7 —

# The Prefrontal Cortex:
# Through Maturation, Socialization, and Regression

Anna Dina L. Joaquin

Human beings are born with an appraisal system that aids in determining the emotional relevance and motivational significance of stimuli received through the sensory systems. The appraisal system determines three kinds of value: homeostatic, sociostatic and somatic (Schumann 1997). Depending on the value, the appraisal system directs appropriate action vis-a-vis motor systems. Homeostatic regulation guides organisms in ways to maintain homeostasis and ensure survival (i.e, to feed, breathe, seek light or darkness, find warmth or coolness). The somatic system pertains to the bodily sensations we experience (i.e. gut feelings). Sociostats are the innate tendencies of a human organism to seek out interaction leading to attachment and social affiliation with conspecifics. Sociostatic value, thus, impels us to seek out interaction with another human being. Lee and Schumann (2005) have proposed that sociostatic value underlies a human being's innate drive to actively pursue social interaction. They have called this drive "the interactional instinct" and find support in the abundance of research in early infant behavioral studies that show infants actively initiating, participating, and sustaining interactions with caregivers (Meltzoff and Moore 1977, 1983; Trevarthen 1977; Tronick *et al.* 1979; See Lee *et al.* 2009 for a review). Ultimately, infants achieve social affiliation and attachment with caregivers who are the source of the language and culture that a child will adopt.

As affiliation and attachment are pursued, caregivers provide a powerful external force that shapes our social knowledge and behaviors through the process of socialization. Though some aspects of human behavior appear to be experience-independent, clearly there are aspects of behavior that are the result of the interactions we have in our social world. In the social sciences, analysts from a language socialization paradigm (Ochs 1988; Ochs and Schiefflin 1984; Schiefflin and Ochs 1986;) have shown through ethnographic work the ways in which "language is used to socialize human beings and how we are socialized to use language" (Schiefflin and Ochs 1986, 163). The perspective holds that from the beginning of social contact, we are socialized to acquire the beliefs, morals, values, and behaviors that are in accordance with the social domains to which one belongs. "The interest is not limited to the role of language in integrating children into society, but is open to investigating language socialization throughout the human lifespan across a range of social experiences and contexts" (Shiefflin and Ochs 1986, 163). Microanalyses of social interactions within normal everyday contexts reveal that socialization is complex, yet also systematic and observable, and that ordinary conversational discourse is a powerful socializing medium through which children learn the ways and worldviews of their culture. Human social behavior is, thus, the product of innate proclivities and socialization.

In the neurosciences, usually through experimental work done under controlled conditions, researchers have been trying to understand the neurobiological underpinnings of social behavior. Using imaging technology that allows us to look at the human brain (i.e. PET, MRI, etc.), researchers have tried to explain social behavior as a physiological phenomenon. Therefore, these two fields with different approaches, foci, and frameworks have been trying to explain interconnected aspects of social behavior: the development of social behavior via language socialization and social behavior as the manifestation of neural underpinnings.

Though both fields have been examining the development of related phenomena and have been making very important contributions to our understanding of social behavior and the process of socialization, they have generally been separate fields with little cross-talk. One objective of this chapter is to integrate knowledge of the socialization practices with what is known about the brain, under the assumption that the methods, frameworks, and findings of each field can be complimentary or be used to inform the other to create a more complete picture of social behavior, socialization, and their neural substrates. Overall, this chapter offers the argument that a society's child socialization practices develop the prefrontal cortex, which afterwards, mediates appropriate social behavior. However, the degeneration of the prefrontal cortex in adults afflicted with diseases such as Frontotemporal Dementia (FTD) results in the opposite trend—the loss of the ability to implement the social behavior that was acquired during infancy, childhood, juvenility, adolescence, and early adulthood. Thus, this chapter looks at the prominent role of the prefrontal cortex in social behavior, and suggests that it is a neural mediator for the processes of socialization. This will be demonstrated by comparing the behaviors of two seemingly different populations in naturally occurring environments. The first population will be children, who have prefrontal cortices that have not fully matured. With ethnographic data, I will show how society's socialization practices work to educate, enculturate, and socialize this part of the brain. The second population, patients diagnosed with FTD, has deteriorating prefrontal cortices, associated with a decreasing ability to implement socialized behavior.

## Maturation of the Prefrontal Cortex

Developmentally, the prefrontal cortex and the lateral temporal cortices develop at a protracted rate in comparison to other regions. Brain regions associated with more basic functions such as sensory and motor processes mature earliest, followed by areas associated with language skills and spatial attention, and then the prefrontal and lateral cortices. Though much of the nervous system develops prior to birth, and though the brain has reached its full size between the ages of 5 and 10, subtle developmental changes occur over a longer period of time. In the months after birth, there is still a continuous explosion of connections between neurons (synapses) followed by a period of stable synaptic density until after puberty when a substantial decline of connections follows (Huttenlocher and Dabholkar 1997). More recent research provides evidence that a wave of synaptic proliferation occurs in the frontal lobes around the onset of puberty (McGivern *et al.* 2002).

Another process involved in neuroanatomical maturation is myelination —the process by which axons are covered with a white fatty sheath of myelin leading to improved conduction and communication between cells. Myelination has been consistently found to dramatically increase during childhood and adolescence. In one MRI study (Sowell *et al.* 1999), the brains of a group of children with an average age of 9, and the brains of another group of adolescents with an average age of 14 were scanned. The results showed a higher volume of white matter in the frontal and parietal cortex in the older children than in the younger group. In study after study, and by different research groups, this linear increase of white matter has been demonstrated (See Blakemore and Choudhary 2006 for references).

Other studies show that there is also a cortical gray matter volume increase in   frontal and parietal regions from early childhood into adolescence. One longitudinal study (Giedd *et al.* 1999) showed that, of 145 healthy boys and girls ranging in age between 4 and 22 years, the volume of gray matter in the frontal lobe increased during pre-adolescence with a peak occurring at around 12 years for males and 11 years for females, followed by a decline in post-adolescence. Research has shown that changes in the frontal regions are especially pronounced and prolonged in adolescence. More specifically, cortical gray matter loss seems to occur earliest in the primary sensorimotor areas and last in the dorsolateral prefrontal cortex (Gogtay *et al.* 2004). Thus, adolescent years still appear to be a time of continued frontal lobe development. Indeed, such findings have been central to arguments regarding the culpability of adolescents who commit crimes and exhibit generally inappropriate behavior (Bower 2004; Scarpa and Raine 2004).

Previous notions of children completely "wired" by the age of 3 have been replaced with the idea that humans undergo a much longer developmental trajectory. Current research suggests that maturation continues well into the teen years, and even into the 20s, with some of the greatest developments occurring during puberty and adulthood (Casey *et al.* 2005). In general, research reveals that this developmental trajectory likely provides a neural substrate for acquiring the skills necessary for higher cognition (i.e. attention, inhibition, perspective taking) and social behavior (Grattan and Eslinger 1991). Such skills are generally a part of the umbrella term, "executive function." Therefore, much experimental research has been aimed at the relationship between the ongoing development of social cognition and the development of the prefrontal cortex.

The Stroop Color-Word Task is a classic measure of frontal lobe function (Adleman *et al.* 2002). In this task, the participant is instructed to name the color of an ink of an incongruent word (i.e. RED printed in yellow ink). Accomplishing this task successfully requires subjects to resolve quickly the cognitive discrepancy and inhibit the incorrect response. In one study, Adleman *et al.* (2002), using the Stroop task on three different age groups (7–11, 12–16, and 18–22), found that the strength of activations in the left lateral prefrontal cortex and the anterior cingulate increases linearly with age, which also occurs in conjuncton with better performance on some measures (i.e. response time) of the task. Another study using the Stroop task on participants between the ages of 6 and 17 years of age focused on the correlation between demographic variables, including age and behavioral performance (Leon-Carrion *et al.* 2004) and found that there was an increase in inhibitory control with age.

While many studies have focused on the development of inhibition, other researchers have looked at emotion recognition. For example, one study shows that adolescents process emotions differently than adults. The study compared 11 to 17 year olds to adults on how they interpret facial expressions (Yurgelun-Todd 2002), and found that the adolescents were not able to correctly identify expressions. For example, when shown a picture with a facial expression displaying fear, only 50% of the teenagers were able to accurately identify the emotion. Adolescents typically identified the emotion as sadness, confusion or shock, while 100% of the adults correctly labeled the expression as fear. Furthermore, brain images reveal that the relative activation of the prefrontal cortex is less than it is in adults. At the same time, the limbic areas (emotional regions) had more activation in the adolescents. Yurgelun-Todd suggests that this may mean that the emotional regions are not yet interacting with the prefrontal cortex in the same way as they do in adults.

Other studies have focused on another function subserved by the PFC—the ability to take another's perspective and make inferences about others' intentions—which has been called Theory of Mind or Mentalizing, and has been shown to have a positive association with social interaction skills (Bosacki and Astington 1999). Given the continuous development of the PFC and the increased complexity of group interactions that adolescents experience, some studies have examined the development of perspective taking in adolescence. In one study (Choudhary *et al.* 2006), the researchers asked 30 pre-adolescents, 40 adolescents, and 37 adults to answer questions that required them to imagine how they would feel in a situation (i.e. You are not allowed to go to your best friend's party. How do you feel?) or how a protagonist would feel in the same scenario (i.e. A girl is not allowed to go to her best friend's party. How does she feel?). The participants were asked to respond to each question by choosing as quickly as possible from one of two emotional faces from a total of five emotional faces. Reaction times showed greater differences among the younger participants than adults. The results suggest that perspective taking in preadolescents and adolescents is developed but is perhaps less efficient than in adults.

In this section, I have provided some of the evidence supporting the claim that the protracted development of the prefrontal cortex may be associated with the increased development of skills, which has been suggested to parallel the development of social behavior. In the next section, ethnographic accounts of children and adolescents in everyday face-to-face interaction, primarily through the framework of language socialization, will demonstrate how an underdeveloped prefrontal cortex may account for some of the behaviors of children and adolescents and how society works vigorously on children and adolescents to teach the behaviors and beliefs that are valued, appropriate, prosocial, and right, and to inhibit those that are not. This next section will show the consequences of an underdeveloped prefrontal cortex on social behavior, and how societies' members, with tremendous effort using complex practices across different situations, act upon the prefrontal cortex to structure its tendencies and values.

## Educating the Prefrontal Cortex

[N]one of the moral virtues arises in us by nature, [R]ather we are adapted by nature to receive them, and are made perfect by habit.

(Aristotle, 29)

Though children are arguably born with some experience-independent tendencies (such as seeking out interaction) and with other innate abilities that are perceived as communicative (Joaquin 2009; Meltzoff 1998; Trevarthen 1977), they are not born with an innate knowledge of what is considered to be socially appropriate and inappropriate behavior. Young children are not born knowing manners, the proper ways of speaking to adults, how to address people respectfully, or how to show concern, compassion, and empathy towards others. Rather, they are born into a social and cultural world where such values are established and can be learned. People's ways of behaving and thinking are not innate traits but are partially a product of the social environment in which they live. Governments, organizations, schools, parents, families, siblings, teachers, coaches, friends—society, work very hard as "teachers" to train and socialize children to the appropriate behavior and morals that reflect those of the culture, family, and organizations (Goodwin 1990; Grusec and Hastings 2007; Hogbin 1970; Ochs and Schiefflin 1984; Paugh 2005; Rogoff 2003). Though explicit instruction to socialize is most common in Western industrialized cultures, even in societies in which listening-in, imitation, observation, and intent participation are the preferred traditions (Crago 1992; Firth 1970; Fiske unpublished manuscript; Hogbin 1970; McPhee 1955), societies' members do not just give children full reign of their upbringing. For example, among the Wogeo of New Guinea:

> The upbringing of the young is not allowed to become a mere haphazard process. The natives have a definite concept of education, for which they use the word *singara*, the primary meaning of which is "steering." Children, they maintain, have to be guided in order to achieve technical knowledge and a proper sense of right and wrong. (Hogbin 1970,142–143)

> The culture is so highly valued, and its mastery by members of the younger generation considered to be so urgent, that the adults take great care to play as prominent a part as possible in its transmission. (Hogbin 1970, 146).

In McPhee's (1955, 84) ethnography of the Balinese, who learn primarily by observation and imitation, corrective feedback is found. For example, the Nengah (musical teacher) generally gazes into space and remains silent, as he models how to play the *gangsa* (a musical instrument), unless to point out a repeated mistake. In other traditional societies, such as the Tikopia, a Polynesian community of about twelve hundred people and free of European influence, there is evidence of socialization. For example, in Tikopia, cleanliness is encouraged by parents. If children are reluctant they may receive "derisive remarks from their companions or elders" (Firth 1970, 81). In another situation in which a daughter was suspected of an "intrigue with a boy of whom she was obviously enamored, the mother threw her down, made uncomplimentary remarks about her morals and beat her in this way" (Firth 1970, 82). Though correcting and enforcing behavior may not always be explicit, members of traditional societies address proper and improper behavior in various ways. Societies' members work especially hard and intervene during the formative years of the prefrontal cortex.

Some attempts to study the socialization of children have been done in controlled laboratory settings, in which samples of infant and child interactions with mothers, fathers, peers (both real and perceived) are observed, recorded and analyzed. However, such studies, by their nature, do not and cannot demonstrate how societies socialize their members in everyday life. As human development is inseparable from social and cultural activities, a person's actions and development can be best understood by observing the interaction in natural social and cultural environments. Ethnography can provide a better picture of how people acquire social knowledge and learn appropriate behavior, and thus can provide a more complete description of how people are socialized into societal and cultural norms. This section uses ethnographic research to show the effects of societal efforts on human social development and social behavior—particularly from a language socialization framework, which has demonstrated that "recurrent speech events" in ordinary face-to-face interactions orient individuals to how to become socially competent members of society (Ochs and Capps 2001). It is important to note that while this chapter's focus is on the role that the social environment has in social development, it does not imply that children are merely passive learners responding to instructions, teaching, and training. Children and adolescents often do not simply comply, but also ask for justification and clarification. Such noncompliance highlights how hard society has to work to foster socialization.

## Inhibition

He, in her analysis of children in a Chinese Heritage Language classroom,[1] found that teachers issued disciplinary directives in response to prior, and often problematic, behavior by students (2000, 131). These directives are not initially formulated overtly. Instead, the problematic behavior is first oriented to and then evaluated, which contextualizes the requested next action from the student, and then is followed by an explicit directive. In this example (7.1 Attention), all the students, except one, are reading aloud in unison with the teacher. The teacher uses a disciplinary directive to encourage the child not

---

1.  All transcripts follow the transcript notations listed in Appendix B. The exceptions are examples 7.1, 7.2, and 7.4. These transcripts were created by the original authors, did not follow the transcript conventions of conversation analysis, and were not altered in this chapter.

```
7.1 Attention

1   Tw: Zhuyi:: you yi ge tongxue::
        attention exist on MSR student
        Attention, there is one student

2       you ti ge tongxue meiyou gen      wo niean a::
        exist one MSR student NEG follow me read
        There is one student who did not read after me

3       Ni  yao bu  nian jiu ji       bu   zhu
        you if  NEG read the remember NEG COMP
        If you don't read aloud you won't remember well.

4       (.3)

5   Tw: Jiu  xue   bu  huei a:
        Then learn NEG COMP PRT
        Then you won't learn

6       Ni kan(.2)beide tongxue dou hen zhuanxin >dui bu dui<?
        You see other student all very attentive correct NEG correct
        You see other students are very attentive, right?

7       (.2)

8       Hao fang xia  shou li      tongxi
        OK  put  COMP hand inside thing
        Now put down the thing in your hands

9       (.2)

10      Kan laoshi.
        Watch teacher
        Look at the teacher.
```

reading along to control himself and to pay attention (2000, 133).

Tw, in line 1, orients the students to the fact that someone is not paying attention and did not follow instructions. Then Tw evaluates the consequences of not paying attention, and again orients the class to the fact that all the other students, with the exception of that one student, are being attentive. In doing this, Tw has already embedded a directive of the proper behavior, which she follows with the explicit directive (line 8 and 10). With this example, He shows how a teacher can use disciplinary directives, in a particular environment, to foster a child's ability to exert effortful control to pay attention.

In another example (7.2 Wait), provided by Bhimji (2002, 99), we can see how family members train younger family members to inhibit their immediate desires. For example, in the following excerpt Alfredo (age 2) wants to play a Nintendo game; however, his cousins (age 8) implicitly and explicitly direct Alberto to be patient.

```
7.2 Wait

1    Daniel:   Vamos a jugar esta.
               Let's play this.

2    Daniela:  Te van a dar horita
               They will give it to you in a little while.

3    Alfredo:  ((Continues to cry))

4    Daniel:   Que espere.
               Wait.

5    Alfredo:  ???

6    Marie:    Que tienes que esperar poquito.
               You have to wait a little.
```

While Alfredo is crying, Daniel in lines 1-2 suggests an alternative game and says *Let's play this*, and offers words of assurance that he will eventually play. Daniel is implicitly directing Alfredo to wait. When Alfredo does not respond appropriately by continuing to cry, Daniel and Marie explicitly state that he has to wait.

Lowi (2007), examined the use of "deontic," or social modals such as *should, ought, would, have to, need to, want,* and *can,* in adult-child discourse in British and American preschools. Such modals are often used in directives to index social responsibility and moral obligation. Lowi showed how, through their deployment, adults socialize children to knowing the next appropriate behavior and how to fulfill social expectations. It should be noted that Lowi also looked at the establishment of gaze and joint attention as part of the structure (Lowi 2007, 109). In all her examples, Lowi observes a recurring interactive structure (Figure 7.1, Lowi 2007, 116) when adults use deontics.

In Example 7.3, Lowi shows how the deontic *need to* with the plural first person pronoun is used with the interactive structure "to indicate the preferred and appropriate responses and actions that are being requested of the child (Liam)" (Lowi 2007, 123); Liam is playing in the sandbox with another child and clearly doing something inappropriate to his schoolmate (Allen).

Prior to this sequence Allen has been in the process of making a sand construction. When Liam enters Allen's play space, Allen immediately demonstrates his objections to Liam's invasive behavior and repeats a number of response cries with variations of *No* and *Stop* (lines 1–6). As Allen is unsuccessful in stopping Liam, Miss B intervenes to get Liam to attend and hear Allen's words and then to regulate himself. Miss B, however, does not employ the same strategy as Allen. Instead, she attempts to get Liam to hear Allen's cries to Stop. She says *Liam can you hear Allen's words*. Miss B uses *can* as a directive for Liam to understand not only the interactive situation, but also

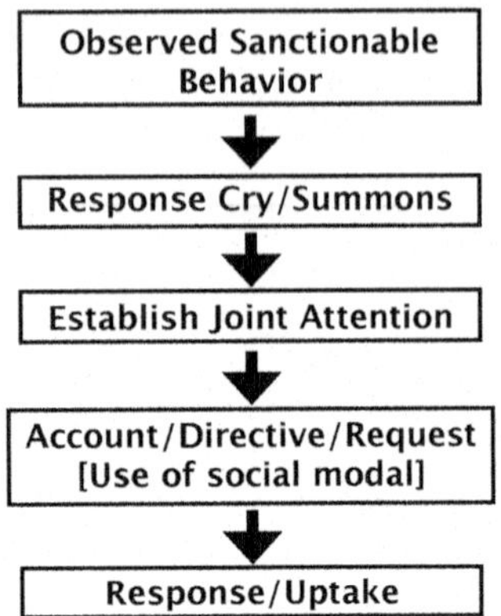


Figure 7.1. Lowi 2007, 116, reprinted with permission

Allen's feelings and, therefore, to get Liam to comply with Allen's wishes. When Miss B's (and Allen's) attempts fail, as Liam continues to play in Allen's space, she takes Liam's arm (line 18) and touches Liam's chin (line 20), while seeking his attention (lines 17 and 18). In doing so, she attempts to reorient Liam's body to a position in which she has his gaze to explicitly assert *Allen does not like that*, and to offer a solution to the conflict. She uses *we need to* to mitigate her directive for the appropriate action. Thus, in this excerpt, achieving the appropriate social behavior requires Liam to understand the perspective of his peer Allen and to inhibit/stop his perseverative behavior.

In this segment, I have shown some of the practices used to teach children to inhibit their socially inappropriate behavior. The Taiwanese teacher employs implicit disciplinary directives, while Alfredo's older cousins use more explicit forms. Miss B uses a range of strategies to achieve joint attention with Liam; she uses multiple sign systems and works hard to alter Liam's ongoing inappropriate behavior. In addition, Miss B demonstrates to Liam that taking the perspective of another person and acting on that understanding will produce socially desirable behavior.

## Perspective Taking and Empathy

As a society, we value attitudes and acts of compassion, sympathy, kindness, and altruistic behaviors. All of these require an ability to empathize with another's feelings and difficulties. However, these qualities are not innately specified. They are in part due to our own personal experience, and are in part encouraged by other members of society. For example, Ahn (2005, 53), in her qualitative study of the strategies teachers used in three child care centers, found that teachers modeled and encouraged children to empathize and show concern for other children:

1.  A girl looks at Seth's hand and blows on his scar.
    Mrs. B tells her, "It's nice of you to worry about his boo-boo."

2.  [A boy falls down and Mrs. S is comforting him].
    Ben comes near the teacher and points at him, "crying, crying."
    Ms. S tells Ben, Yes, he's crying. He is sad.
    He may be afraid. Sometimes we even get scared when we fall down.
    Thank you for your concern. I think concern for others is a big boy
    thing to do!

Ahn (2005, 53)

```
7.3 We Need To Go Over There
Allen=4 yr. old, Miss B=Preschool teacher

01  Allen:     No. Nooooo. No! Stop that(.)Stop!
02             Sto:p tha:t! Sto::p Sto:::p!
03                 ((Allen tries to move Liam's hands))
04             Sto::p!
05                 ((Allen looks up for assistance))
06             Sto:::p! No:!
07  Miss B:    Liam can you hear Allen's words?
08             Liam what is he saying?
09             Liam, [Liam,
10                 ((Liam does not respond))
11  Allen:          [stop!
12  Miss B:    Liam, [What is Allen [saying?
13                 ((Liam continues playing with sand))
14  Allen:          [stop           [stop
15             Stop Stop Stop Stop Sto::p
16                 ((Liam continues to be unresponsive))
17  Miss B:    Liam,


18             ((Miss B moves and
               takes Liam's arm))


19             Liam. Listen, Li- Liam
20             ((Miss B touches
               Liam's chin))
21             Allen doesn't like that

22             ((Liam looks up at Miss B))
23             We need to go over there




24             and play where Allen wants you to play
25             Al- this was Allen's=
26             =you come play down here. ((pats bench))
27                 ((Liam moves down))
```

These two examples demonstrate how teachers validate children's display of empathy by indicating that their actions are the right responses. Though it is unclear in example 2, whether Ben is in fact showing concern by pointing to the boy who is crying, Ms. S treats Ben's actions as a display of empathy and rewards him.

He provides yet another example of how teachers encourage understanding of others (2000, 132). In example 7.4, the students are writing words on the blackboard, while the teacher is watching. B2 (Weiwei) is writing so big on the blackboard that he is writing into a classmate's (Liyin's) space. To orient B2 to the problem, Ts comments on the size of B2's writing (line 1). B2 looks at Ts as if he is confused (line 2), displaying that he does not understand the import of Ts's comment. Ts then continues to evaluate the consequence of the size of B2's writing (line 3). As the problem is evaluated, B2 demonstrates that he understands the problem  (line 4) and that his appropriate next course of action is to erase what he just wrote. Only after B2 has changed his behavior is the explicit directive made (line 5). In Excerpt 7.4 (below), He provides a situation in which a disciplinary directive is used to foster in a child "the idea that one should show concern for others" (2000, 132).

Interaction with peers is also seen as important in the development of empathy in Japanese preschools. So for example, Tobin *et al.* (1989, 35) observed that teachers encouraged 4 and 5 year olds to "adopt" 1 or 2 year olds. Thus, the researchers frequently observed older preschoolers helping younger children take off their shoes and outdoor clothing and go up and

```
7.4 Write Smaller
B2/Weiwei=Student; Ts-Teacher

1   Ts:     Weiwei zi  xie   de hao  da  o!
                Character  write      very big PRT
                How big is Weiwei's writing!


2           ((B2 turns to look at Ts questioningly))


3   Ts:     Zheme da  Liyin jiu  bu  gou     difang le=
                This  big        CONJ NEG enough place  PRT
                If you write this big, Liyin will not have enough space


4   B2:     =Oh-oh::  ((erasing what he just wrote))


5   Ts:     Ok  xie  xiao   yidian   la.
                Write small a little PRT
                Ok, write a little smaller.


6           ((B2 writes again, in smaller size))
```

down stairs. In fact, children often accept special charge of younger ones, and they even help change and feed the infants. One of the teachers stated that: "[W]e feel this contact with babies and toddlers gives them a chance they might not otherwise have to develop empathy (omoiyari) and to learn how to anticipate the needs of others (ki ga tsuku)" (Tobin *et al.* 1989, 35).

The role of seemingly dispreferred peer interaction (e.g. fighting) is also seen as important in becoming empathic and a "good" citizen of society. For instance, one of the Japanese teachers commented that:

> When children are preschool age they naturally fight if given the chance, and *it is by fighting and experiencing what it feels like to hit someone and hurt them and to be hit and be hurt that they learn to control this urge to fight*, that they learn the dangers of fighting and get it out of their system.
>
> (emphasis mine; Tobin *et al.* 1989, 33)

Thus, across cultures, there are ways in which interactions within the family, schools, and with peers teach the value of understanding others' emotional states and the necessity to act upon that understanding.

In this section, we have looked at instances in which children and adolescents are not attentive, speak at inappropriate times, perseverate in their inappropriate behaviors, are impatient and want immediate gratification, show lack of insight to another person's perspective and only consider their own, and so on, *unless* someone intervenes and teaches/socializes appropriate behavior. Children are simply not born with a complete system of social knowledge nor, in some cases, an inclination to acquire one.

Paugh has even examined how children are socialized to work-related values and expectations as they participate and listen to their parents' conversations and narratives about work. Through overhearing their parents, children get a "glimpse into their parents" perspectives on work—what it takes to be boss...positive qualities of an employee, and that there are parameters for when and how people work" (2005, 68). Goodwin also notes how the telling of "instigating stories" among peers about violations of social expectations and the resulting righteous indignation toward such acts, also "function to suggest future courses of action" for the hearers (1990, 267). And as Ochs and Capps (2001) state, such narratives about personal experience elaborately encode and perpetuate moral worldviews. Personal narratives

> generally concern life incidents in which a protagonist had violated social expectations. Recounting the violation and taking a moral stance towards it provides a discursive forum for human beings to clarify, reinforce, or revise what they believe and value. (Ochs and Capps 2001, 45–46)

Though this reference relates to work, it is a generalizable statement about how views and attitudes are formed in children. In each of the examples in this section, parents, teachers, and peers attended to a violation of social behavior, and took a moral stance toward it. In doing so, they made an effort to bring the behavior to the forefront and gave the violators an opportunity to take note of their interlocutors' moral stances, the effects of their actions, and the opportunity to either reinforce or revise what they believe to be the right or wrong behavior.

I have shown with experimental and ethnographic research how suboptimal prefrontal cortices may account for some of the inappropriate behavior in typically developing children and how society's members may act as external prefrontal cortices to socialize children to prosocial behavior. Further evidence of the intrinsic role of the prefrontal cortex in the process of becoming a socially competent member of society can be found through individuals who have incurred prefrontal damage or developed, a neurodegenerative disease known as Frontotemporal Dementia, creating impairments in affect, empathy, perspective taking, inhibition, and self control—aspects of social cognition that are highly valued, and as we have seen, taught and reinforced in society.

### Effects of Early Prefrontal Damage on Socialization

Some evidence of the effects of early prefrontal damage on social behavior comes from two patients who suffered from bilateral prefrontal damage early in life. The first is G.K. who, because of an increased head circumference during the first 7 days of his life, had bilateral ventricular punctures to remove hematoma fluid resulting in bilateral prefrontal lobe lesions. Records from multiple sources revealed "that serious behavioral difficulties were first identified by the age of 8 yrs. He did not respond to parental discipline, always sought gratification and his immediate needs [and] never developed adequate friendships" (Price *et al.* 1990, 1384). Only under firm guidance and two school transfers was he able to graduate from high school. Records also show that he joined the Marine Corps, but was dishonorably discharged after only six weeks of service. Over the next ten years after graduating from high school, G.K. was imprisoned eight times on charges of assault, forgery, grand larceny, and lewd behavior. He was also charged with arson of two pubic buildings and masturbating in public. Other examinations showed that he was overly "impulsive," and "showed little insight or empathy."

The second patient is M.H., who at the age of four was hit by an automobile, also resulting in bilateral frontal lobe damage. Over the next year, observers noted that, "she hit her brother—cut her sister with glass. Family members lived in constant terror and once called the police when she threatened them at knifepoint. She repeated first and second grades, and was only successful with special tutorials" (Price *et al.* 1990, 1385). When she was 17 years old, she was raped while wandering through a local cemetery, and even returned to the scene on another day only to be raped again by the same man. Though M.H. received individual psychotherapy and medication, her behavior did not significantly change.

G.K. and M.H.'s behavior is even more striking in contrast to their siblings. G.K. was the eldest of six brothers. Though one suffers from mild retardation, the other four siblings are college graduates, and one is a lawyer. His father was a successful landscaper and his mother was a nurse. The family environment was not observed to be particularly stressful or chaotic. As for M.H., she is the fourth of six children. None of her five siblings had similar behavioral problems. Her father was an optician and her mother is employed as a purchasing agent. Neither family had a history of psychiatric disease. In households such as these, G.K. and M.H. would not have been socialized to behave in the ways they did, but their behavior was rather the consequence of early frontal damage.

Marlowe (1992) reported the case of P.L., who, at three years old, incurred an injury in the right prefrontal cortex from a lawn dart. Though he recovered from the injury, within weeks after his surgery, behaviors that were previously absent became evident. He was aggressive, impulsive, and hyperactive. In pursuit of his own desires, he would act-out and show no remorse for his actions. Eventually P.L. was given some counseling and efforts were made to teach him strategies to stop and evaluate his behaviors. However, such intervention was ineffective. Unfortunately, there have been several cases of anecdotes and records like P.L., M.H., and G.K. (Ackerly and Benton 1948; Anderson *et al.* 1999; Powell and Voeller 2004).

Previous developmental notions suggested that an earlier onset of brain damage had a more likely chance for recovery than brain damage incurred as an adult because an immature brain is more capable of considerable plasticity and reorganization of function (see Benton and Tranel 2000 for a review). This notion was supported by some studies in which individuals with early damage to language areas seemed to show very few speech and language impairments as adults. This trend, with the exception of a few notable cases (Eslinger *et al.* 1997), however, does not appear to be the case with early onset damage to the prefrontal cortex. In fact, early onset damage may have consequences that are "considerably more grave than patients with adult-onset lesions" (Tranel and Eslinger 2000, 274). Early prefrontal damage results in individuals who are unable to be socialized to acceptable, advantageous, and moral behavior. This research is consonant with the notion that the process of socialization described builds prefrontal circuits that support appropriate social and personal reasoning and prosocial behavior.

## Effects of Adult Prefrontal Damage on Socialization

Cases in which *adults* incurred prefrontal damage have been documented as well. What is interesting, although somewhat predictable, about such patients is that though they act in ways that are socially deviant, unlike the children with early damage, they actually possess and can access under controlled conditions their "social knowledge." Thus, these individuals have internalized the social knowledge and rules to a certain degree, yet prefrontal damage, whether it be the result of surgery or a tragic accident, has reversed the forces of socialization. This effect is demonstrated through experiments similar to those conducted with children as well as anecdotal evidence.

The ventromedial (VM) prefrontal cortex is often associated with impairments in emotional expression and social conduct. Hornak *et al.* (1996) conducted a study comparing 12 subjects with damage restricted only to the ventral part of the frontal lobe to 11 subjects with damage outside the frontal lobes or in the dorsolateral prefrontal region or the posterior lateral surface. In the first part of the study, they showed photographs of facial expressions (i.e. sad, angry, frightened, disgusted, surprised, happy, and neutral) to patients with damage to the ventral part of the frontal lobe. Patients were shown one photograph at a time and asked to choose from a list of adjectives that best described the photograph. The second part of the study involved patients listening to a tape with emotional sounds that were chosen to reflect sadness, anger, fear, disgust, puzzlement, satisfaction and neutral affect. They were then asked to name each sound from a list. In addition to the testing, subjects were asked questions that would reveal their awareness of their emotional ability. In general, in both the facial and vocal identification tasks, patients with VM damage were severely impaired in their ability to correctly identify emotional stimuli, whereas the non-ventral group was very minimally impaired, and were in fact not significantly different than the normals. A follow up test showed that several of the members of the ventral group did not have any problems in either a face recognition or an environmental sound identification test. Some patients were even able to imitate and produce sounds expressing emotions, though they were not able to identify them.

Another study examined only the ability to comprehend facial expressions in patients with the temporal variant of frontotemporal dementia (tvFTD), a subtype of FTD that involves the amygdala and anterior temporal lobes asymmetrically as well as portions of the OFC (Rosen *et al.* 2002). Emotional comprehension was evaluated by showing photographs of female faces depicting emotional expressions. Subjects were asked to 1) discriminate between the identity of two faces, 2) discriminate between two emotions, 3) name emotions depicted, 4) select a photograph displaying an emotion requested by a researcher, and 5) match a depicted emotion with the same emotion. As hypothesized, patients with tvFTD performed poorly compared to controls in all five subtests. Such a deficit in interpersonal skills can have consequences for real world behavioral competencies. One study found that VM damage not only resulted in severe emotional impairment, but that it accounted for impairments in real world competencies as well (Anderson *et al.* 2006).

Some researchers have also used the Interpersonal Perception Task to assess the ability of patients with lesions in the orbitofrontal and/or the dorsolateral regions to understand social interactions (Mah *et al.* 2004). The Interpersonal Perception Task requires subjects to make judgments on different aspects of relationships of the persons depicted in scenes. The scenes are authentic and are excerpts from real-life social situations. The researchers modified the task so that participants assessed kinship, intimacy, competition, social status, and deception by perceiving the nonverbal aspects of social exchange (i.e. facial expressions, gesture, and body torque). Social titles (e.g. mother) were omitted from the scenes. In this way, subjects are supposed to "read between the lines" of verbal dialogue and interpret nonverbal cues (Mah *et al.* 2004, 1250). For example, a scene in which two women and a man are shown conversing with each other is shown to a patient, and the patient is asked "which woman is engaged to be married to the man?" The study found that patients with orbitofrontal cortex (OFC) lesions performed poorly compared to the control subjects. In addition, the study also showed that patients with primarily dorsolateral prefrontal cortex (DLPFC) lesions performed significantly worse in the task. It was also found that there was a correlation between the extent of the damage in the dorsolateral area and poorer perception ability.

The same researchers (Mah *et al.* 2005) administered the Test of Social Intelligence to patients with VM and DLPFC lesions and normals. The test includes a series of drawings and cartoons that require subjects to use nonverbal cues to interpret social and emotional situations. The first task presents subjects with drawings of hand gestures, body postures, and facial expressions that show the same thought or expressions. Subjects are then given four alternative drawings from which they must choose one that expresses the same emotion as the preceding drawings. In the second task, subjects are instructed to choose one of four alternative cartoon panels to complete a series of panels depicting a social interaction. The third task requires subjects to interpret the meaning of verbal statements in different social contexts. Lastly, the subjects are shown a cartoon panel with the final panel missing. Subjects must choose the correct panel from three alternatives that depict the event that would follow, based on the characters emotional reaction to a situation. Thus, this task requires the subject to interpret the intentions and feelings of characters in social situations. Consistent with their previous research and as Mah *et al.* (2005) hypothesized, VM patients had lower scores than the controls. Patients scored particularly low in the tasks that required them to name an emotion expressed through facial expressions, gestures, or body posture or to construe the intentions and feelings of characters. These studies are consistent with the vast amount of literature showing deficits in socially relevant behavior following VM lesions.

Impairments in reading social cues are important for inferring other's mental states and the significance of their actions. This ability may be called theory of mind, or an awareness of the mental states of others and the implications for their motives and intentions. Though studies show that theory of mind is not diminished in patients with VM damage and that they are still able to complete first and second order false belief tasks as well as normals, they demonstrate difficulty in more complex tasks (Stone *et al.* 1998; Torralva *et al.* 2007). One task is a faux pas test, in which subjects read a story that may or may not contain a social faux pas committed by one of the characters. This test is useful in that to understand that a faux pas has occurred subjects have to represent two mental states, that of the person committing the faux pas who is unaware that they have said something inappropriate, and that of the person hearing it who might feel hurt or offended. Children between the ages of 9 and 11 usually pass this test. In another task, the "mind in the eyes" task, subjects are shown photographs of the eye region of faces, and are then required to choose a word that best describes what the person in the picture is thinking or feeling (Torralva *et al.* 2007). In both tasks, patients with frontal lobe damage performed significantly worse than controls.

In another study, Gregory *et al.* (2002) compared the performance among patients with FTD in the VM area, patients with Alzheimer's disease, and normals. Participants were given first- and second-order beliefs tests, faux pas detection, and reading the "mind in the eyes" tasks. As hypothesized, FTD patients had significant impairments in theory of mind, while Alzheimer's patients failed only the second order belief task, which places heavy demands on working memory. FTD patients performed particularly poorly on the faux pas test and the "mind in the eyes" test. Another interesting finding was that there was a striking concordance between the ranking of patients according to the degree of their impairment on theory of mind tasks and the severity of frontal lobe atrophy. Thus, studies have supported the notion that FTD patients are impaired in their abilities to empathize and take the perspective of another.

Other studies have also reported that patients with lesions in the orbitofrontal and ventromedial prefrontal cortex show a lack of concern for social and moral rules. J.S. is a notable case, reported by Blair and Cipoloti (2000). He was a 56 year-old man, who worked as an electrical engineer and one day experienced trauma in the right frontal region. After his injury he had deficits in maintaining social norms. He was also reckless regarding others. On one occasion he continued to push around a wheel-chaired patient despite the patients screams of terror. He showed a lack of remorse and regret when he hit nurses. He showed impairments in empathy and had "profoundly disturbing social interactions" (2000, 1124–1125). Blair and Cipoloti gave J.S. a number of cognitive tests and compared the results to five inmates of Wormwood Scrubs prison with psychopathy. In comparison to the inmates, J.S. showed a "profound impairment on expression recognition and emotional responding tasks." He also showed impairment in attributing fear, anger, and embarrassment to others. He also "failed to discriminate transgressions which result in victims and those which result in social disorder and to judge inappropriate behaviors likely to induce anger in observers" (2000, 1134).

Experimental studies provide valuable information about what skills related to social behavior are impaired by FTD and other damage to the prefrontal and temporal regions. Anecdotes give general insight to the effects of FTD as well. Reliance upon them may have been necessary because the long-term consequences of such social deficits are difficult to capture. It is difficult to record a person making bad economic decisions and their ramifications, which may come instantaneously or over an extended period of time. Such descriptions and anecdotes may provide an incomplete picture of how such a disease affects the daily lives in mundane social situations. Thus, in the next section, FTD patients in every day situations are examined to show how this disease affects the comportment, inhibition, decision-making, and attentional abilities that society has invested in to develop in its members.

### Another Lens

A general description of FTD in the literature is that patients act in ways that are comparable to children. Indeed, the literature and anecdotes mentioned above on prefrontal damage describe patients who seem to have regressed in their social skills and behavior, even though they retain knowledge of the rules of social behavior. This general description is further supported by ethnographic research on FTD patients.

What will be shown in the following sequences are FTD patients behaving in ways that warrant the deployment of directives by their spouses, and other participants, to inhibit and control them. The first participant involves "Romeo," who at the time of data collection was 63 years old. He is a former adult school teacher and has been married to his wife "Juliet" for over 20 years. He was diagnosed with FTD in early 2006 with reported behavioral changes beginning several years before.

In this first example (7.5 Hold off), Romeo (ROM) and Juliet (JLT) have been creating a prayer box for Romeo to put in all of his written prayers. The activity in itself is suitable for a child, as the prayer box is a shoebox that Juliet wanted Romeo to cover and decorate by taping on some colorful construction paper. Andrea (AND), the ethnographer, has been helping Romeo, but Juliet is now helping him with the activity.

While Juliet is talking to Andrea, Romeo prematurely tapes a piece of construction paper to the box resulting in her scolding Romeo and saying his name multiple times, showing her annoyance, and telling him that he is jumping ahead (lines 6–7), because the cover has to be either written or printed on the computer first. Though Romeo acknowledges Juliet's scold (line 8), while Juliet continues to work on the cover, he gets a piece of tape.

```
7.5 Hold off
Romeo, 15 February, 2007C

01   JLT     and that's the sort of::: hot pink. But>anyway<
02   ROM     hh
03   JLT     ugh hh
04   AND     [well color]s kinda tricky for=
05   ROM     [now what   ]
06   JLT     =aw Romeo Gaw h Romeo >Romeo Romeo Romeo Romeo:
07           <your jumpin ahea:d.
08   ROM     okay.
09           (1.2)  ((gets piece of tape from dispenser))
10   JLT     hey lets: just hold off hold off oka:y
11              ((places hands on Romeo's))
12   ROM     [okay] ((gets tape))
13   JLT     [hold]off [hold off]
14   ROM               [okay    ] now what?
15   ROM     what?
16   JLT     hold off (.) Do you want-Romeo. Do you want Romeo's

17           pra:yer- Romeo stop for a second.



18   JLT     Do you want Romeo's pra:yer bo:x (.)


19           to be ha:nd printed
             or from the computer?
20   ROM     From the computer.
               ((Places tape on box))
21   JLT     I guess I ain't gonna be able
22           to stop him (.) he's ready to finish.
```

Juliet again scolds Romeo with multiple utterances of the directive hold off (line 10) and places her hand on Romeo's to symbolically show Romeo to stop. Again he acknowledges Juliet's scold as if he was going to listen to her, but against her directions he still gets a piece of tape (line 11). Juliet then begins to ask Romeo what he wants on the cover. However, Romeo anxiously leans in to attempt to place the piece of tape that he has in his hand. Juliet then gives him a direct order to *stop for a second*, accompanied with a hand gesture that definitively indicates "no" (line 16). Despite, her repeated efforts to control Romeo's behavior, she is unsuccessful. In the end, she concedes and says *I ain't gonna be able to stop him* (lines 21–22).

In this sequence, Romeo is provided a range of systematic resources including language structure, prosody, and gesture so that he can participate in a common course of action in an appropriate manner (Goodwin and Goodwin 2004). However, though showing markers of compliance to Juliet's directions (e.g. okay), Romeo does not inhibit himself and perseverates with his desire to tape the cover. Though Romeo's perseverative behavior initially may not be a social failing, his repeated noncompliance to her repeated directives and displays of disapproval show his inappropriate behavior.

In the next excerpt, the FTD patient is "Kelly" who has a Ph.D. in piano performance and is a former piano teacher. She is married to "Bron." In 2003, she began to exhibit behavioral changes and since then has been rapidly declining in her cognitive and emotional abilities. She was first diagnosed with manifestations of FTD in 2005 (see Torrisi Chapter 2). The following sequence captures her lack of inhibition, which results in social sanctioning from her coparticipants. Kelly (KLLY) and Bron (BRON) are eating at a restaurant with two ethnographers (AND and LISA), and are sharing their wine tasting adventures.

In excerpt 7.6, below, the participants have been engaging in talk about wine, when Bron produces the story preface *I remember*—(line 8) to tell about a time when he was in Sardinia. As he gives background information, Kelly unexpectedly reaches over him to grab a glass of wine that is to his left. In response to her impulsive behavior, Lisa laughs (line 13 and 16), and Bron reprimands her and gives a directive to control her urge (line 15), while Andrea provides a reason why Kelly should not be reaching over for the wine (she has had two already) (line 18). The three different responses from three different participants index the social violation, and suggest that Kelly's behavior is, at least within this context, deviant.

The two examples cited in this section display Romeo and Kelly acting upon an urge that their co-participants "work" to inhibit, through directives, various linguistic forms, and gestures.

While other neurodegenerative diseases, such as Alzheimer's, rob patients of their memory, FTD is often considered the disease that robs patients of emotions—not only of the ability to display their own, but also the ability to understand the feelings of others. This is painfully clear in instances when an intimate is displaying intense emotional pain, and an FTD patient is co-present. In these situations, the patient often does not behave or respond in a way that shows any sign of empathy, concern, or attempt to understand. Prior to excerpt 7.7 (So much pain), Juliet has been talking about how she has been coping with her back pains and other difficulties in her life. Copresent are Romeo (who is sitting in the arm chair to her right), and an ethnographer (Andrea), who is sitting on the floor across from both Romeo and Juliet.

In line 1, Juliet says that she doesn't know how to run her life and what she should do next, and then starts to cry. At the end of her turn she turns her gaze to Romeo, who is already looking at her, and thus identifies him as the next speaker. Though they are mutually gazing at one another, Romeo turns away, gets up and walks to the kitchen to get *more coffee* (line 6). Though providing an account for his leaving is an appropriate social cue, his exit follows a

```
7.6 Reach Over
Kelly, 13 March, 2007B

01  KLLY    California's the wine capital of the U.S.
02  AND     it is: for sure
03  LISA    France is very upset about that so::
04  AND     uh h
05  LISA    the fact that the US is [competitive in wine
06  BRON                            [>Of course some of those
07          places you have to be um:: sort if a little bit
08          adventurous I: remember that I was at one of the
09          place in Sardinia (0.2) d uh:: (.) you know I was
10          just looking at some of the wines and some of the
11          wines were ?? bottles but there I was staying with
12          an Italian fa[mily] and:
13  LISA                 [hhh ]

14  KLLY    Give me a taste.
15  BRON    O::: o:: o:: wai::t a mi:nu:ute.
16  LISA    hhh
17  KLLY    [??
18  AND     [You've had two already
19  BRON    h hhh
20          (5.0)

21  BRON    And I told them about the wines
22          [that I wanted to buy
22  KLLY    [give me a little sip
23  BRON    and they said that's not the way to do it. And then
24          he took to the bar the local bar and then behind the
25          bar there was this huge bottle of wine
26  AND     ha ha ha ha ha
```

moment in which his gaze and physical orientation would seem to be a display of availability as a possible co-participant (Kendon 1985) and yet his next action and utterance actually indicate otherwise. While Romeo is out of the room, Juliet launches a pre-telling of a story with *the most upsetting thing happened to me on Sunday*, which will give an example of one thing that she has had to deal with recently. As Romeo walks back into the room and prepares to sit, she continues with a crying voice the pre-telling of an event that happened to her on Sunday. Situated within her pretelling is an assessment of the event, which Andrea follows with a continuer (line 13), showing her collaboration with Juliet in the assessment (Goodwin and Goodwin 2004). Juliet, though, still does not go into the story, but continues to build up the story that she is about to tell with a question marked with a crying voice as she says *Have you ever had something happen to you that you wondered why they were happening?* (lines 14–15). Andrea, in response to the question, shows agreement, *Mhm*, and displays that she can empathize with Juliet. Juliet then launches her story with background that includes a description of the physical pain she was experiencing at the time as she describes that she was in **so** much pain. Her facial expression also shows that the pain was excruciating. Along with the sniffles and description, she has also become more emotional. While Andrea continues to display her participation as a listener (line 20), Romeo shifts his gaze away, reaches for a hat on the couch to his right, puts it on his head, and then reaches for a piece of paper in front of him and starts to read. After coughing and drinking some water, Juliet restarts her story by providing more background. At this point, Romeo's head is completely turned away from Juliet and he continues to read the piece of paper.

Despite Romeo's physical position as a participant in this framework and the multiple displays from Juliet (crying voice, sniffles, facial expressions, and descriptors) that solicit a collaborating response from her hearers, Romeo behaves in a way that seems as if he does not have any concern for his wife. In fact, he seems disinterested and unsympathetic. His behavior is particularly noticeable in contrast to Andrea, who is showing signs of listening, understanding, and empathy, which is also highlighted by the researcher's offer of a tissue (line 24).

In another example (7.8 Can you play this for me?), Romeo, Juliet and Andrea have just come home from the pharmacy. When Juliet tried to pay for the prescriptions, she was told that her insurance has been terminated. The following conversation takes place in the car on the ride home from the pharmacy. Juliet is driving, Romeo is in the passenger seat, and Andrea is in the backseat, while Juliet is talking about the situation (lines 4–12), noting that this is one thing she needs as much as a *hole in the head*. Andrea shows that she understands Juliet's circumstances as evidenced; she provides agreement tokens (lines 13 and 17), and even concludes Juliet's turn with an appropriate

```
7.7 So Much Pain
Romeo 12 December, 2006 (*=crying voice)

01   JLT     I don't know how to run my life.
02           (2.0)
03   JLT     tch .h* sometimes I'm so overwhelmed I don't even
04   JLT     know (1.0) what I should do ne:xt.


05           (8.0)
06   ROM     more coffee
07           (4.2)


08   JLT     I'm trying to take it (1.6) one thing at a ti::me
09           (0.2) but (6.2) I had (3.2) tch the most upsetting
10           (2.3) thing happen to me on Sunday,
11           (4.0) ((Romeo walks back into the living room))
12   JLT     *.tch I don't know why it happened.
13   AND     m:::
14   JLT     have you ever had something happen that you wondered
15           theyre happening?
16   AND     Mhm
17   ROM     ((clears throat))
18   JLT     *I was in- (1.2) ((sniffles)) I was in s::- I was in
19           so much pai:n
20   AND     Mhm


21           (2.6)
22   JLT     *we went to church tch.
23           (2.2) ((Juliet coughs twice, clears throat, drinks))
24   AND     You need a tissue?
25   JLT     ((shakes head 'no.'))
```

description of the consequences that would result if Juliet's insurance were terminated (bills would be coming at her left and right) (line 19). Juliet confirms Andrea's assessment of the situation by her repetition of *left and right* (line 20), which also shows that Andrea is aligned with Juliet. Beginning from line 23, Juliet's tone changes from angry to emotionally distraught as she begins to cry and says that she does not need *one more thing* to happen to her. Her repetition of *one more thing* emphasizes her emotion and indicates her view that many things have been happening to her that have made her life very difficult. At a point when Juliet is very emotional, Romeo makes a request, *An-, can you play this for me on the thing.* Romeo's behavior is striking in comparison to Andrea, who is not family, as opposed to Romeo who is her husband, yet Andrea is the one who is actively listening and providing tokens of understanding, and systematically showing that she is a hearer of the talk (Goodwin and Goodwin 2004), while Romeo remains relatively silent, not showing any sign of concern or empathy toward Juliet.

The behavior demonstrated in these examples reflects how FTD affects a

```
7.8 Can you play this for me?
Romeo, 17 January, 2007T (*=crying)


01   JLT      Andrea
02            (0.8)
03   AND      yeah
04   JLT      they said my insurance was not active
05            (1.0)
06   AND      (You need more help)
07   JLT      I kno:w that (0.4) the owner (0.2) of the business
08            (0.1) who covers it has been screwing around with it.
09   AND      m:::
10   JLT      and I know that heez been tryin to (.) uh:: make a
11            cha::nge in some peoples pla::ns and he assured me
12            mine was no:t affected
13   AND      m h[m: ]
14   JLT         [Now] (0.4) heez I need one more thing like I need
15            a hole in th head you know that if it was inactive
16            (.) for that surge[ry (.) that bills are gonna be
17   AND                        [ye:ah
18   JLT      coming at me::
19   AND      left and right
20   JLT      left and right so::::: unbelievable you just don't
21            even know
22   AND      yeah
23   JLT      *i- i- i- just don't know why all this is happening
24            to me I just don't know why:: I get stuck with one
25            more thing and one more thing that is not of the
26            normal (.) why do things keep coming at me I don't
27            know [(*
28   ROM          [An- An- can you play this for me on the thing?
29            (.)
30   JLT      Nobodys there Romeo
31   ROM      kay
32            (1.4)
33   JLT      I don't understand (   ) *its too much (.) for
34            one person to take
35   AND      yeah
```

patient's capacity to understand others and/or to act upon that understanding in a way that is appropriate, which are highly valued behaviors that are taught to children.

## Conclusion

In this chapter, I have shown that society's child socialization practices and the development of the prefrontal cortex are intertwined. An underdeveloped prefrontal cortex is associated with less executive function and therefore, to some extent, socially undesirable behaviors observed in children and adolescents. However, as ethnographic studies show, vigorous socialization practices of parents, caregivers and peers educate, socialize, and enculturate the prefrontal cortex with the values and behaviors that are socially acceptable, and afterwards that brain region continues to mediate appropriate social behavior in adults. Although, just as socialization results in the acquisition of social knowledge, this chapter also shows that damage to the prefrontal cortex, or having a disease such Frontotemporal Dementia, results in the opposite—the loss of the ability to implement social behavior that was acquired during infancy, childhood, adolescence, and early adulthood. Thus, the prefrontal cortex has a prominent role in the development and maintenance of social behavior.

## References


Ackerly, S. and A.L. Benton.

  1948  Report of a case of bilateral frontal lobe defect. *Research Publications: Association for Research in Nervous and Mental Diseases* 27: 479–504.

Adleman, N., V. Menon, C. Blasey, C. White, I. Warsofsky, G. Glover and A. Reiss.

  2002  A developmental fMRI study of the Stroop Color-Word task. *Neuroimage* 16: 61–75.

Ahn, H.J.

  2005  Child care teachers' strategies in children's socialization of emotion. *Early Childhood Development and Care* 175(1): 49–61.

Anderson, S.W., J.Barrash, A. Bechara and D. Tranel.

  2006  Impairments of emotion and real world complex behavior following childhood- or adult-onset lesions in ventromedial prefrontal cortex. *Journal of the International Neuropsychological Society* 12: 224–235.

Anderson, S.W., A. Bechara, H. Damasio, D. Tranel, and A. Damasio.

  1999  Impairment of social and moral behavior related to early damage in human prefrontal cortex. *Nature Neuroscience* 2: 1032–1037.

Aristotle

2004 *Nicomachean Ethics.* Montana: Kessinger Publishing.

Benton, A. and D. Tranel.

2000 Historical notes on reorganization of function and neuroplasticity. In *Cerebral organization of function after brain damage,* edited by H.S. Levin and J. Grafman, 3–23. New York: Oxford University Press.

Bhimji, F.

2002 "Dile Famile": Socializing language skills with directives in three families in South Central Los Angeles. Unpublished Dissertation, University of California Los Angeles, Los Angeles.

Blair, R.J.R. and L. Cipolotti.

2000 Impaired social response reversal: A case of "acquired sociopathy." *Brain* 123: 1122–1141.

Blakeslee, S.

2008 *A disease that allowed torrents of creativity.* The New York Times.

Blakemore, S.J., and S. Choudhary.

2006 Development of the adolescent brain: Implications for executive function and social cognition, *Journal of Child Psychology and Psychiatry* 47 (3/4): 296–312.

Bosacki, S. and J.W. Astington.

1999 Theory of Mind in preadolescence: Relations between social understanding and social competence. *Social Development* 8(2): 237–255.

Bower, B.

2004 Teen brains on trial. *Science News* 165(19): 291.

Casey, B.J., N. Tottenham, C. Liston and S. Durston.

2005 Imaging the developing brain: What have we learned about cognitive development? *Trends in Cognitive Science* 9(3): 104–110.

Choudhury, S., S. Blakemore and T. Charman.

2006 Social cognitive development during adolescence 1: 165–174.

Crago, M.

1992 Communicative interaction and second language acquisition: An Inuit example. *TESOL Quarterly* 26(3): 487–505.

Eslinger, P., K. Biddle and L.M. Grattan.

1997 Cognitive and social development in children with prefrontal cortex lesions.

In *Development of the prefrontal cortex: Evolution, neurobiology, and behavior,* edited by N.A. Krasnegor, G.R. Lyon and P.S. Goldman-Rakic, 215–335. Baltimore, MD: Paul H. Brookes.


Firth, R.

1970 Education in Tikopia. In *From child to adult: Studies in the Anthropology of Education,* edited by J. Middleton, 75–90. New York: The Natural History Press.

Fiske, A.P.

nd (unpublished manuscript) *Learning a culture the way informants do:Observing, Imitating, and Participating* Unpublished manuscript, University of California, Los Angeles.

Geidd, J., J. Blumenthal, N. Jeffries, F.X. Castellanos, H. Liu, A. Zijdenbos, T. Paus, A. Evans and J. Rapoport.

1999 Brain development during childhood and adolescence: A longitudinal MRI study. *Nature Neuroscience.* 2(10): 861–863.

Gogtay, N., J. Giedd, L. Lusk, K. Hayashi, D. Amyeenstein, A. Vaituzis, T. Nugent, D. Herman, L. Clasen, A. Toga, J. Rapoport and P. Thompson.

2004 Dynamic mapping of human cortical development during childhood through early adulthood. *Proceedings in the National Academy of Sciences* 101(21): 8174–8179.

Goodwin, M.H.

1990 *He Said-She Said.* Bloominton: Indiana University Press.
2006 Participation, affect, and trajectory in the family directive/response sequences *Text and Talk* 26(4/5): 513–542.

Goodwin, M.H. and C. Goodwin.

2004 Participation. In *A Companion to Linguistic Anthropology,* edited by A. Duranti, 222–244. Maldan, MA: Blackwell.

Grattan, L. and P. Eslinger.

1991 Frontal lobe damage in children and adults: A comparative review. *Developmental Neuropsychology* 7: 283–326.

Gregory, C., S. Lough, V. Stone, S. Erzinclioglu, L. Martin, S. Baron-Cohen and J. Hodges.

2002 Theory of mind in patients with frontal variant frontotemporal dementia and Alzheimer's disease: theoretical and practical implications. *Brain* 125: 752–764.

Grusec, J. and P. Hastings, eds.

2007 *The handbook of socialization: Theory and research.* New York: The Guilford Press.

He, A.

2000 The Grammatical and interactional organization of teacher's directives: Implications for socialization of Chinese American children. *Linguistics and Education* 11(2): 119–140.

Hogbin, H.I.

1970 A New Guinea childhood: From weaning till the eighth year in Wogeo. In *From child to adult: Studies in the Anthropology of Education,* edited by J. Middleton, 134–162. New York: The Natural History Press.

Hornak, J., E.T. Rolls and D. Wade.

1996 Face and voice expression identification in patients with emotional and behavioural changes following ventral frontal lobe damade. *Neuropsychologia* 34(4): 27–261.

Huttenlocher, P. and A. Dabholkar.

1997 Regional differences in synaptogenesis in human cerebral cortex. *Journal of Comparative Neurology* 387: 167–178.

Joaquin, A.D.L.

2009 Interactional readiness: Infant-caregiver interaction and the ubiquity of language acquisition. In *The Interactional Instinct: The Evolution and Acquisition of Language,* edited by N. Lee, L. Mikesell, A.D.L. Joaquin, A.W. Mates and J.H. Schumann, 108–150. Oxford: Oxford University Press.

Kendon, A.

1985 Behavioural foundations for the process of frame attunement in face-to-face interaction. In *Discovery strategies in the psychology of action,* edited by G. Ginsburg, M. Brenner, and M. von Cranach, 229–253. London: Academic Press.

Lee, N. and J.H. Schumann.

2005 *The Interactional Instinct: The evolution and acquisition of language.* Unpublished manuscript, Los Angeles.

Lee, N., L. Mikesell, A.D.L. Joaquin, A.W. Mates and J.H. Schumann.

2009 *The interactional instinct: The evolution and acquisition of language.* Oxford: Oxford University Press.

Leon-Carrion, J., J. Garcia-Orza and F.J. Perez-Santamaria.

2004 Development of the inhibitory component of the executive functions in children and adolescents. *International Journal of Neuroscience* 114(10): 1291–1311.

Lowi, R.

2007 *Building understanding through language and interaction: Joint attention, social modals and directives in adult-directed speech to children in two preschools.* Unpublished Dissertation, University of California Los Angeles, Los Angeles.

Mah, L., M. Arnold, and J. Amyafman.

2004 Impairment of social perception associated with lesions of the prefrontal cortex. *American Journal of Psychiatry* 161: 1247–1255.

2005 Deficits in social knowledge following damage to the ventromedial prefrontal cortex. *Journal of Neuropsychiatry* 17: 66–74.

Marlowe, W.

1992 The impact of right prefrontal lesion on the developing brain. *Brain and Cognition* 20: 205–213.

McGivern, R.F., J. Anderson, D. Byrd, K.L. Mutter, and J. Reilly.

2002 Cognitive efficiency on a match to sample task decrease at the onset of puberty in children. *Brain and Cognition* 50(1): 73–89.

McPhee, C.

1955 Children and music in Bali. In *Childhood in contemporary cultures,* edited by M. Mead and M. Wolfenstein, 70-98. Chicago, IL: Chicago University Press.

Meltzoff, A. and K. Moore.

1977 Imitation of facial and manual gestures by human neonates. *Science* 198(4312): 75–78.

1983 Newborn infants imitate adult facial gestures. *Child Development* 54: 702–709.

Meltzoff, A.

1998 Infant intersubjectivity: Broadening the dialogue to include imitation, identity and intention. In *Intersubjective Communication and Emotion in Early Ontogeny,* edited by S. Braten, 47–62. Cambridge: Cambridge University Press.

Ochs, E.

1988 *Culture and language development: Language acquisition and language socialization in a Samoan village.* Cambridge: Cambridge University Press.

Ochs, E. and B. Schiefflin.

1984 Language acquisition and socialization: Three developmental stories. In *Cul-*

*ture theory: Essays on mind, self, and emotion,* edited by R.A. Shweder and R.A. Levine, 276–320. Cambridge: Cambridge University Press.

Ochs, E. and L. Capps.

2001 *Living narrative: Creating lives in everyday storytelling.* Cambridge, MA: Harvard University Press.

Paugh, A.

2005 Learning about work at dinnertime: Language socialization in dual-earner American families. *Discourse and Society* 16(1): 55–78.

Powell, K. and K. Voeller.

2004 Prefrontal exective function syndromes in children. *Journal of Child Neurology* 19: 785–797.

Price, B., K. Daffner, R. Stowe and M. Mesulam.

1990 The comportmental learning disabilities of early frontal lobe damage. *Brain* 113: 1383–1393.

Rogoff, B.

2003 *The cultural nature of human development.* Oxford: Oxford University Press.

Rosen, H., R. Perry, J. Murphy, J. Kramer, P. Mychack, N. Schuff, M. Weiner, R. Levenson, and B. Miller.

2002 Emotion comprehension in the temporal variant of frontotemporal dementia. *Brain* 125: 2286–2295.

Schieffelin, B. and E. Ochs.

1986 Language Socialization. *Annual Review in Anthropology* 115: 163–191.

Schumann, J.H.

1997 *The Neurobiology of Affect in Language.* Los Angeles: Blackwell.

Scarpa, A. and A. Raine.

2004 The psychophysiology of child misconduct. *Pediatric Annals* 33(5): 296–304.

Sowell, E.R., P.M. Thompson, C.J. Holmes, R. Batth, T.L. Jernigan, and AW. Toga.

1999 Localizing age-related changes in brain structure between childhood and adolescence using statistical parametric mapping. *NeuroImage* 6: 587–597.

Stone, V., S. Baron-Cohen and R. Knight.

1998 Frontal lobe contributions to theory of mind, *Journal of Cognitive Neuroscience* 10: 640–656.

Tobin, J., D. Wu, and D. Davidson.

1989 *Preschool in three cultures: Japan, China, and the United States.* New Haven, CT: Yale University Press.

Torralva, T., C. Kipps, J. Hodges, L. Clark, T. Bekinschtein, M. Roca, M. Calcago and F. Manes.

2007 The relationship between affective decision-making and theory of mind on the frontal varient of fronto-temporal dementia. *Neuropsychologia* 45: 342–349.

Tranel, D. and P. Eslinger.

2000 Effects of early onset brain injury on the development of cognition and behavior: Introduction to the special issue. *Developmental Neuropsychology* 18(3): 273–280.

Trevarthen, C.

1977 Descriptive analyses of infant communicative behavior. In *Studies in mother-infant interaction,* edited by H.R. Schaffer, 227–270. London: Academic Press.

Tronick, E., H. Als and L. Adamson.

1979 Structure of early face-to-face communicative interactions. In *Before Speech,* edited by M. Bullowa, 349–370. Cambridge: Cambridge University Press.

Yurgelun-Todd, D.

2002 *Inside the teenage brain.* Retrieved September 20, 2007, from http://www.pbs. org/wgbh/pages/frontline/shows/teenbrain/.

# — 8 —

# Dispassionate Heuristic Rationality Fails to Sustain Social Relationships

Alan Page Fiske

> FTD is a model to understand morality and the brain. FTD patients retain knowledge for moral behavior and the ability to make "rational" moral judgments. [But] FTD patients commit sociopathic acts. (Mendez 2006)

This chapter proposes three interconnected theses. The first is that the behavioral variant of frontotemporal dementia is the result of loss of social motives and moral emotions, while other non-social motives and emotions and most other components of cognition remain intact. The second thesis is that the heuristics and biases of human reasoning make it impossible to sustain meaningful social relationships in the absence of social motives and moral emotions. Social motives and moral emotions are adaptations that evolved because they enable people to sustain important relationships. Studies of the conversations of FTD patients, together with participant observation, demonstrate what happens when social motives and moral emotions fade away. The analyses of the neurobiology of these patients reveals that intrinsically motivated relationships cease to function when the right orbitofrontal cortex and right temporal pole degenerate.

## The Social Relationships of Dispassionate Rational Actors

The behavioral (right predominant) variant of frontotemporal dementia (FTD) is a disease of social relationships (Clark *et al.* 1986; Mendez *et al.* 1996; Jagust *et al.* 1989; Neary *et al.* 1998).[1] Diagnostic criteria for FTD character-

---

1.    It is a continuing joy and intellectual adventure to working with the authors of the

ize it in terms of features that include

> "early loss of social awareness (lack of social tact), early signs of disinhibition (e.g., unrestrained sexuality)…emotional unconcern (indifference, lack of empathy, apathy)…animia (inertia, aspontaneity)…progressive reduction in speech (economy of utterance)." (Lund and Manchester Groups 1994)

Some of the consensus diagnostic features are formulated in terms of "early decline in interpersonal conduct, early impairment in regulation of personal conduct, early emotional blunting…aspontaneity and economy of speech, press of speech." (Neary *et al.* 1998)

Family members often report that patients become lazy, irresponsible, and untrustworthy. Or they cease to attend to others' needs, while freely indulging their own desires (Mendez and Cummings 2003; Mendez *et al.* 1996). Their families say that they are unaffectionate, and uncaring, without 'warmth' (Miller *et al.* 2001). Often their supervisors fire them, most of their friends abandon them, and their spouses may divorce them. They squander joint checking accounts or they fail to complete their work. According to his brother Fred, the apathetic patient Ned had been a driven, "anally" organized man, self-disciplined in his finances, in working out and in diet. After he developed FTD he stopped working out, gained a lot of weight, and played golf instead of going to work at his management job. So he was fired and had to take a similar, lower level position with a smaller organization. But he failed to do that job, too, and after a couple of months was fired again. His wife divorced him (Fiske Sept. 10, 2008: field notes).

But while this is happening, patients continue to be "rational": during the early stages of the disease their cognitive and perceptual skills remain largely intact, they generally recognize what others think and feel, and they understand the consequences of their actions. Generally in the first years their knowledge and memory are largely intact. Moreover, perhaps the most

---

chapters in this book, Lisa Mikesell, Andrea Mates, Michael Smith, Netta Avineri, Sam Torrisi, Anna Joaquin, and John Schumann. My thanks to them for help and comments on earlier drafts of this chapter, too. Sven Waldzus also provided incisive, valuable comments. This book grew out of the Social Relations in FTD Project, whose tireless, congenial, stimulating team consists of Brian Ellis, Sabrina Pagano, Brett Erzinger, Laura Loriga, Matthew Gervais, Jiro Tanaka, and Keziah Conrad. Jill Shapira provided enthusiastic, insightful guidance getting us started, and her compassionate commitment to the patients has been a model for us all. Most fundamentally, this entire project depends on the gracious cooperation and endless education that Dr. Mario Mendez continues to provide us. Thank you, Mario, for your openness to our social science and humanities perspectives, and above all, for entrusting your patients to us. We thank the UCLA Faculty Senate and the Association for Frontotemporal Dementias for invaluable seed grants. What a team, what a collaboration!

mysterious feature of FTD is that patients do not recognize that anything is wrong. They are not aware that they have lost their social motives and moral emotions. How is this possible? How can a person cease to feel love and compassion, cease to experience embarrassment or guilt, and cease to have a sense of fairness or responsibility, without noticing the change? As Avineri (this volume) points out, faced with persistent questioning, a patient may concede that she has memory problems, but few patients recognize that they have become amoral or asocial. When the neurologist pushes a patient, Louise, to say what problems she has beyond failures to remember, Louise turns to her daughter Jess for help answering the question. Louise recognizes that her daughter might be able to answer the question, but she herself is not aware that anything else is wrong—and indeed she steadfastly denies that she has any problems other than difficulty remembering things.

An FTD patient in the early years typically does not lack a self: she apparently has a clear representation of who she is—but her representation corresponds to the way she was *before* the onset of the disease. The disease commences and progresses, but it seems that she does not update her representation of herself—despite the manifold censorious reactions she persistently provokes in others. She ignores her frequent offenses and grievous transgressions. The changes in her behavior are striking to others, but she is somehow blind to them.

So what is wrong with FTD patients? Why do their social relationships disintegrate while they remain dispassionately rational?

It is nearly impossible to answer this question using interviews, verbal tests, or paper and pencil instruments, because in the first years of FTD, patients tend to act more or less normally in the clinic, and they commonly score in or near the normal range on most standard neurological tests. And in PET, SPECT, or MRI images, behavioral variant patients show right ventrofrontal and/or right anterior temporal degeneration. Because of their lack of insight and failure to update their self-concept after the onset of FTD, patient self-reports are nearly useless as measures of actual motives, emotions, or current behavior. Patients say they are just fine; they have no complaints, perceive few, if any, changes in themselves, and report that they are living a normal life (see Avineri, this volume). But their family members give a completely different account. So to find out what is going wrong, we need to observe how patients interact in everyday life in natural settings. This is what we are doing in the Social Relations in FTD Project. The research reported in this book stems from the first participant observation and video and audio recordings of the social relationships of FTD patients in their real, everyday worlds.

The Social Relations in FTD Project has four objectives. Our first and most immediate aim is to understand how and why people afflicted with behavioral variant of FTD distress and offend the people they interact with, while the patients themselves are content and oblivious. The goal is to observe first-hand the aberrations that actually constitute the disease. These aberrations are much more salient in the patients' everyday lives than they are in the structured, limited interactions of the clinic. A scientific account of anything must be based in the first place on careful, systematic observation and precise description of the natural phenomenon, but FTD had never been directly observed outside the artificial constraints of the clinic. So the SRFTD team is, in the first place, performing the foundational function of the naturalist.

Our second aim is to understand the nature of rational actors. The dominant theory in the social sciences posits that normal people are rationally self-interested actors, except where emotional biases or cognitive limitations interfere with rational decisions. We believe that FTD patients in the early stages of their disease show us how dispassionately rationally self-interested actors really behave—dysfunctionally. What links these two first aims is our theory that FTD patients lack social motives and moral emotions. We theorize that social relationships have no intrinsic meaning for them, so they interact purely instrumentally, using relationships only to obtain non-social ends. Most normal people, we believe, engage in social relationships largely because good relationships are inherently meaningful and intrinsically rewarding (Fiske 1991, 2002).

Our third goal is simply the converse of the second: to elucidate the role of emotions and motives in sustaining social relationships. One aspect of this is to transcend the prevalent approach to human action, and therefore to psychopathology, which we regard as methodologically individualistic. We believe that, ironically, FTD will help us understand the nature of social relationships as structured dynamic interaction which cannot be reduced to the psychological properties of the individual participants.

Our fourth aim is to understand the neurobiology of social relations, especially relational motives and moral emotions. We theorize that the core of FTD is the degeneration of the regions of the brain that motivate people to seek, sustain, and repair relationships—the neural systems that make relationships emotionally rewarding. When these brain systems deteriorate, patients lose the motives they once experienced as liking, love, respect, pride and responsibility. When these neural systems cease to function, people apparently also cease to experience moral emotions such as empathy, compassion, shame, embarrassment, guilt, remorse, moral outrage, or envy. FTD is the result. In contrast, we theorize that FTD patients retain non-social motives: they show no apparent decline in hunger, sexuality, curiosity, frustration, or fear. Freud's obsolete psychoanalytic concepts provide a surprisingly concise metaphor, in which one could describe FTD as the loss of the superego, while the id remains intact and the ego remains frozen in time. In a more modern conceptualization, FTD consists of the loss of the neural systems that evolved for the specialized function of complex, nuanced human social relationships, while the phylogenetically older systems that subserve the asocial lives of most mammals continue to function. We believe that FTD is informative about the neural systems that subserve the emotional and motivational bases of social relationships.

This book presents the pioneering work of the applied linguists in the Social Relations in FTD Project, relying primarily on conversation analysis (CA). Before we launched the Social Relations in Frontotemporal Dementia Project, all that was known about FTD was how they behaved in the clinic, the structure and histology of their brains, and what family members said about them. The Social Relations in FTD Project incorporates CA because CA provides precisely grounded descriptions of the interactions with FTD patients that are distressing to their interlocutors. While CA explores the proximate acts that sustain and coordinate interaction from moment to moment, classical CA does not often go very far toward analyzing the psychological mechanisms or long-term social relational consequences of utterances. But CA describes the details of everyday communication, and these details can be analyzed to understand the eventual causes and consequences of conversational actions or inactions. Some previous CA research has demonstrated how meaningful interaction is maintained despite neurological impairments that degrade conversational capacities (Goodwin 2003; Goodwin *et al.* 2002). In this chapter I do just the opposite, showing how neurological impairment of the lower right front of the brain degrades social relationships. This chapter draws on the CA of the applied linguists in the project, whose chapters characterize precisely how FTD patients' conversational interactions break down. I put the CA together with our participant observation and video ethnography, which permits us to illuminate the emotional and motivational causes of that breakdown, together with the social relational consequences of these interactive malfunctions. CA tells us precisely what happened; participant observation provides first-person experiential reports of how patients' interlocutors—especially the ethnographers themselves—reacted and adapted to what happened.

The first section of this chapter reflects on the CA and ethnography from this book and some of our other observations to argue that the core deficit of FTD patients is their loss of social motives and moral emotions, while their other motives and emotions remain intact. The second section of the chapter briefly deals with epistemology, addressing the problem of how we can know others' motives and emotions. This problem is especially difficult in FTD, since patients themselves *report* that they still have moral emotions and social motives that they consistently fail to demonstrate in their current social behavior. The third section briefly discusses our epistemological strategy of using multiple, maximally diverse methods to provide convergent evidence about FTD, social motives and moral emotions. The fourth section presents a theory for why dispassionate human rationality is insufficient to sustain functional, meaningful social relationships.

## Ftd Patients' Deficits in Social Motives and Moral Emotions

### *My mind was elsewhere*

When in the presence of people one knows, speakers in the US are expected to collaborate to sustain a conversation. Unless participants are busy with activities that require concentration, or have been in each other's presence for a long period (such as on a long walk or drive), it is polite to keep talking, avoid prolonged silences, and ask questions or introduce new topics when necessary to sustain the conversation. Failing to sustain a conversation is awkward because it implies that one has no wish to interact, and thus does not want to sustain a relationship. Beyond simply keeping the conversation going, in middle class American culture, asking people questions about themselves and their lives generally conveys a somewhat higher level of "interest," respect, and desire to be connected. (In other cultures asking personal questions can be seen as intrusive, aggressive, or as an attempt to control or be dominant.) Not asking how someone is, what they are doing, and so forth suggests a lack of empathy—it suggests that the speaker does not care about the other.

When I interviewed Ned, the 57-year old apathetic FTD patient, he initiated new topics only four times in an hour, three of which were requests for a drink of water. A few times I intentionally stopped speaking for up to two or three minutes, letting the conversation die. These are extremely long pauses for face-to-face interactions in which participants are not engaged in any other activities. He remained attentive but showed little or no discomfiture at the silences. Although I knew this was characteristic of FTD patients, particularly apathetic ones, I got frustrated after a while trying to "fill" the time and began to feel slightly desperate as I hunted for ways to keep the interaction "alive." I asked him many questions about his interests, activities, and life, to most of which he replied "I'm not sure."

When Andrea first met the apathetic patient Romeo, she reported that Romeo seemed "odd:" "Most of his oddness was in his lack of initiation toward me as a stranger, and his lack of extending talk" (Mates, Nov. 20, 2006: field notes). Andrea reported that to have conversations with Romeo, she had to ask lots of questions, but "he gives short, relatively unsatisfactory answers" (Mates, Aug. 22, 2007: field notes; also Mates, Jan. 24, 2007: field notes; discussed in Mikesell 2009a). When Matt went to meet Romeo nine months later he knocked on the door; Romeo opened the door, paused, said "Hi"—and then walked away to watch TV. Matt's field notes remark: "He asked no questions of me. He followed up no questions with extensions. Like a robot!" (Gervais, Aug. 9, 2007: field notes). According to his wife, Romeo was chatty and engaged before he developed FTD. Even the disinhibited patient Kelly virtually never asks the ethnographers a question (Torrisi, Chapter 2, this volume).

Pilot analyses of recordings show that interlocutors conversing with Steve and Romeo initiate new topics several times in 30-minute samples of conversations, while Steve and Romeo never initiated new topics in these samples. This is not simply because people make special efforts to draw FTD patients into the conversation: in pilot analyses of recordings of normals interacting with normals, topic initiation is common. There are even greater differences between FTD patients and normals in rates of asking questions: Pilot analyses show that the interlocutors of Steve, Romeo, and Kelly ask both personal and impersonal questions at rates that are 5 to 20 times higher than the average rates of the three FTD patients, regardless of whether the rates are calculated per minute or per word.

Note that patients are not expected to ask clinicians personal questions, or even to sustain the conversation; the clinician generally directs the interaction by asking questions, giving advice, or requesting cooperation ("Please look at this and tell me…"). Hence FTD patients' failures to ask questions and sustain conversations would not be readily apparent in that setting.

Steve typically gives minimal answers, often one-word: "yes," "mhmm," "good," usually without expansion (Mikesell 2009b). Sometimes he answers with an affirmation or negation when a fuller answer is conversationally required. For example, asked what he's reading in the newspaper, he replied "I don' know," and when asked if he knows what his daughter's husband does, he simply answers, "mm hmm." When asked if he's ready to read the comics out loud as a dialog, he agrees he's ready, but then doesn't read. Bron reports that he no longer asks Kelly questions about herself, because she long ago ceased to respond to such questions (Torrisi, Chapter 2, this volume).

In short, the patients do not hold up their end of the conversations, leaving their interlocutors to do all the conversation "work." Further, patients did not ask the ethnographers or others about themselves. This made the ethnographers uncomfortable: being with the FTD patients felt awkward. The ethnographers reported that they often felt ignored and disrespected.

When someone speaks to an FTD patient, the patient often repeats what the first person said: Sam says, "You could describe it," and Steve replies, "Could describe it, yes" (Mikesell 2009a Chapter 6). While these responses answer the literal question, they fail to respond to the conversational demands for a more elaborated personal reply, and hence may be perceived as ungracious and uncooperative. In some contexts normals reply with this kind of repeat to claim primary rights to information to which their interlocutor has claimed rights (Stivers 2005). In a sample of conversations involving Steve and Romeo, they respond with these modified repeats to 14 of 51 (28%) yes-no interrogatives, while the others present respond to none of these yes-no questions this way. Looking at declarative utterances, Steve and Romeo give modified repeats as agreements to 21 of 32 (66%) statements, compared to a rate of 1/82 (1%) for their interlocutors (Mikesell 2009a Chapter 6). Steve, whose disease was more advanced, uttered more repeats than Romeo, and Romeo uttered more of these repeats as his disease progressed. These full response repeats of FTD patients may be aggravating to the interlocutors of FTD patients, who may perceive them as surly or argumentative.

Beyond speech, the desire to relate to someone is expressed by staying with them—simply being in their presence. FTD patients sometimes fail to stick around. For example, Kelly frequently leaves to check her medicine schedule, and Romeo often gets up in the middle of a conversation and leaves the room to get himself coffee. One time, Anne reported that when preparing to take the dog for a walk together, Anne put Steve's hat on him and then went out of the room to get something. While she was doing this, he simply left without her (Torrisi, Aug. 13, 2006: field notes). As we noted above, when Matt came to meet Romeo, Romeo left him at the door and returned to his TV.

There are social consequences of FTD patients' failure to sustain conversations or show interest in their interlocutors by initiating topics, asking personal questions, or elaborating answers. These deficits make their interlocutors feel ill at ease and unwanted. All but the most loving and committed family members may be discouraged from trying to engage with FTD patients, with the result that patients' relationships with coworkers, their friendships, and their family relations may attenuate or cease. Who wants to hang out with someone who never engages, who never cares what you are saying, who doesn't even care whether you talk to them or not? These aberrations may not be apparent in the clinic, where the patient is continuously responding to the clinician (see Avineri, Chapter 5, this volume). The patient in the clinic does not need to take initiative to sustain the conversation by introducing new topics, and clinicians do not expect patients to ask them personal questions. In this setting, unlike most others, it is often appropriate to give a short, unelaborated response.

### What's it to me?

FTD develops insidiously; for a while at first, the afflicted person retains many social capacities. Mates remarks early on, "Like Steve, Romeo also has marked prosodic features that seem to carry emotional meaning on them which by extension enters him into social space. He is not just spouting propositions, affirming or denying some other proposition. He is evaluating and responding" (Mates, Nov. 28, 2006: field notes). As time passed, however, Romeo's prosody seemed to gradually wash out so that his speech flattened. The second time she visited Romeo, Mates helped him choose photographs for an album. She reports that she found the experience of interacting with him "not only affectively flat, but even alienating" and "off-putting" (this volume). Similarly, in response to a question, Ned told me flatly, without any expression, that his parents had died—his mother just five months ago, he said. He did not respond to my effusive condolences (Fiske, Sept. 10, 2008: field notes). Compassion, along with self-conscious concern to present oneself as a caring person, move people to show concern when people are in need, and to care for them if possible. Driving in the car one day, Anne, Steve, and Sam listened to an NPR report of an African woman who died because her surgeons refused to complete a cesarean section when they learned her insurance would not cover the cost. Torrisi exclaimed in horror and Anne cried. Steve laughed and did not react to Anne's tears (Torrisi, Jan. 19, 2006: field notes). Some FTD patients sometimes do respond to others' expressed emotions in ways that are situationally appropriate in the moment, and some, like Steve, frequently smile and nod responsively in the early stages of their disease. But these preserved responses seem to be "directly" and "automatically" elicited by facial expression, posture, or voice tone, and they seem to be immediate and transitory, with little effect on any prolonged course of action. Many FTD patients, however, do not respond to even the most obvious emotional needs of others, regardless of whether others' needs could be anticipated from experience or are directly communicated.

Participants joining in everyday social interactions implicitly commit to a modicum of mutual compassion and mutual aid—in relational models terms, a low intensity communal sharing relationship (Fiske and Haslam, 2005). Torrisi and Mikesell's chapters (Chapters 2 and 4, this volume) each present a videotaped moment when the patient Kelly, her husband Bron, Sam, and two care-facility staff members, Elinor and Rachel, are meeting around a table. An assistant, Gina, arrives with a tray of six glasses of water; as she sets down the tray she spills all the water onto the table. While everyone else responds, Kelly simply watches impassively, continuing to eat her cookie, then tries to get up to leave to check her medicine schedule. Her failure to make any effort to help clean up and her failure to help repair Gina's face are violations of basic politeness norms; her disinterest conveys a lack of empathic compassion required by the communal sharing model that organizes being together in this event.

In a videotape, we see Juliet tell Andrea about a very upsetting experience at church, saying how overwhelmed she is and how helpless she feels, unable to understand why so many bad things are happening all at once. She weeps. Sitting next to them, Romeo utterly ignores Juliet, continuing to eat breakfast and recite prayers he routinely reads (Joaquin, Chapter 7, this volume; 12 Dec. 2007 video). This is typical of Romeo, as we can see by the fact that Juliet is addressing Andrea, not Romeo. FTD patients may not respond to even the gravest of crises. When Fred and Ned's father lay dying, Fred reports that he called Ned's wife to send him to come see their father before he died (Fiske, Sept. 10, 2008: field notes). Ned flew in, arrived at the house where their father was on his death bed, and flopped down and turned the TV on without asking about their father or going in to see him. This appalling breach convinced Fred that there was something seriously wrong with Ned, impelling him to bring Ned in for a neurological consultation.

Such failures make FTD patients seem callous and cold, or seem no longer to love their families, and may eventually motivate others to avoid continuing to attempt to relate to them. Most of the daily signs of FTD are not dramatic, merely abrasive: mundane rudeness, everyday disregard for others' sensitivities, and failure to be moved by others' distress. Co-workers, friends, and family members may endure these bleak signs of FTD for years before seeking a clinical consultation, feeling hurt and rejected all the while. Furthermore, these deficits are not likely to be apparent in the clinic, where the focus is on the symptoms, concerns, and needs of the patient. Patients in a neurology or psychiatry out-patient clinic are rarely called upon to show sympathy, to behave compassionately, or to help anyone.

### *No offense taken*

Like many apathetic FTD patients, Steve, Romeo, and Louise show very, very little initiative. But while they rarely initiate action, they are quite responsive to commands. So their family members constantly tell them what to do. At home on video in front of Andrea, Juliet tells Romeo precisely how to put a paper cover on his own prayer box and, when he starts before she thinks he should, commands him to "Stop!" taping it down (Joaquin, Chapter 7, this volume; Feb. 15, 2007C video). He shows no sign that these task assignments, precise instructions, or commands annoy him. Steve typically seems not to want to do anything. But like Romeo, he tends to be compliant, although he often fails to completely follow a command that requires execution of several steps. Sometimes he expresses verbal irritation or non-verbal resistance to these directives, but often he complies without showing signs of being offended (e.g., Torrisi, July 26, 2006 and Aug. 1, 2006: field notes;

also discussed in Mikesell 2009a, Chapter 4). At one point Torrisi asks him if he wants to get up, and he says he does not. But when Torrisi *tells* him to get up, he does so. Ordinarily it would be inappropriate for a much younger guest to tell his older host what to do, but Steve shows no sign of irritation (Torrisi, July 17, 2006: field notes; also discussed in Mikesell 2009a). Kelly is a piano teacher, but she is not visibly upset when Bron says he has indefinitely rescheduled all her piano lessons (Mikesell, Chapter 4, this volume). When Louise states to Dr. Mendez that she isn't having any problems, she placidly accepts her daughter Jess's correction that she forgets things, gets confused, and presently doesn't remember that her hearing aids are not working (undated video recording, first week of October 2003). Neither being contradicted nor being labeled forgetful and confused in front of Dr. Mendez, and on video, seem to bother her at all. Right after these corrections she unabashedly—and, conversationally, quite unnecessarily—volunteers and then lingers on not remembering Dr. Mendez until she saw him again (Avineri, Chapter 5, this volume).

Perhaps these family members always gave these patients a lot of directions or corrections before the onset of their FTD. It seems unlikely, but we don't know. However, adults often are upset by affronts to their dignity, and even when they are used to a spouse incessantly giving directions, people may show annoyance. The FTD patients we have observed display little concern about being bossed around. These patients seem to lack pride, not feel humiliated by their loss of status, and not feel embarrassed at being ordered around in front of acquaintances or even strangers. It seems as if they do not take offense because they do not *feel* offended.

### No reason to be embarrassed

Although Steve is a good pool player and presumably still knows the rules, he does not follow the rules or even take turns (Torrisi , July 17, 2006: field notes; also discussed in Mikesell 2009a, Chapter 4). Ordinarily, a person overtly breaking the rules of a game would frame the breach as a joke or nonplay of some sort, or would be emotionally concerned about (and prepared for) the other player's anger. Steve seems not to care how Sam will react. Many FTD patients' conversations become less flexibly adapted to the situation, disregarding the flow of discourse; their speech becomes progressively more stereotyped as they use a limited repertoire of utterances repeatedly. This may reflect damage to systems that are more specifically linguistic, especially ones in the left anterior regions of the prefrontal cortex, rather than the right anterior systems that are more social relational. But perseverative stereotyped utterances imply a social defect, as well. This is most notably illustrated in our experience by Kelly, who repeatedly tells people scripted stories about her abortion and her brother's suicide (Torrisi, Chapter 2, this volume). She told these stories to the ethnographers soon after they meet her, making them feel uneasy. But she showed no evident shame or embarrassment, and the very fact of her telling these stories to new acquaintances suggests a lack of shame or embarrassment.

Romeo does a number of things that make people uncomfortable. Mates reports that he eats her popcorn without asking, spits repeatedly while they are out walking, fans his crotch, picks his nose, and smells as if he has not wiped himself properly (Nov. 13, 2007: field notes; cf. McKhann *et al.* 2001, 1804). Normally a sense of prospective embarrassment prevents people from doing such things, but Romeo does them, and does not seem to be embarrassed. Mikesell (Chapter 4, this volume) cites a staff member's report that Kelly defecated in a wastebasket. As Mikesell mentions, one woman in the UCSF FTD documentary reports that her husband changes clothes in his open cubicle at work. Another woman in the documentary reports that her husband sits outside for hours killing and counting ants. Apparently these patients lack the self-consciousness—the concern about others' comfort or judgments—that would prevent most people from doing these things.

FTD patients often have compulsions, perseverating in the performance of specific acts when there is no functional point in doing so (Boone *et al.* 1999; Mikesell, Chapter 4, this volume). These acts, like the ant-killing and counting, often involve excessive checking or pointless enumeration. For example, Kelly constantly goes to her room to check her medication schedule, and Romeo incessantly asks Andrea to turn the TV on and off (Julia has forbidden him to touch the controls himself), interspersed with trips to the kitchen to reheat coffee (Mikesell, Chapter 4, this volume). Vera very frequently says, "It's a wonder of the world," and other FTD patients also repeat stereotyped phrases. FTD behaviors such as this resemble the obsessive thoughts and the compulsions, including checking and counting, that characterize obsessive-compulsive disorder patients. But OCD patients are ashamed of their compulsions, so they usually make great efforts to conceal their compulsions, even from family members and close friends, and sometimes from their own therapists. In contrast, FTD patients are not self-conscious about their compulsions, and make no attempt to hide them.

FTD patients also lack any shyness or reserve, often approaching, speaking too, and even touching strangers, or touching acquaintances in ways that invade their personal space. For example, in a store, Vera speaks to and touches a stranger, calling him "a little munchkin" (Smith, Chapter 3, this volume; video Dec. 11, 2003A). She often approaches strangers on the street and engages them in conversation, making them uneasy but showing no sign of embarrassment, herself (e.g., video Nov. 23, 2003A). Lack of self-conscious embarrassment or shame may reduce an FTD patient's inhibitions, releasing actions that are distressing to others. But patients who lack embarrassment, shame, or pride may also be exceptionally compliant if they consequently lack any concern about their dignity, and hence placidly follow anyone's instructions without getting their feathers ruffled. Sometimes in social interactions with family or co-workers, FTD patients' meekly undemurring obedience may partially make up for lack of initiative and failure to follow-through. Nonetheless, it is an ominous sign in the context of the other mundane changes described by the conversation analysts in this volume.

### Crimes and misdemeanors

FTD patients rarely perceive the changes in their emotions and behaviors, and if they do perceive the changes at all, they don't care about them. Their behavior in the clinic, their cognition and memory are typically fairly normal in the early stages, so there are no definitive tests for FTD. This also means that descriptions of FTD are largely based on reports of family members who bring them to the clinic. These reports naturally tend to include accounts of dramatic, egregious transgressions and especially bizarre actions, and indeed the decision by family members to insist that a patient come to the clinic often seems to be precipitated by a dramatic social breach or a series of major norm violations. When the family member gets to the clinic they often are faced with the challenge of persuading the clinician that there really is something drastically wrong with the afflicted person, despite the person's more or less benign, cooperative behavior, their unremarkable account of themselves, and their lack of any complaints. So family members are likely to recount dramatic or bizarre transgressions; if they do not, the clinician may fail to be sufficiently impressed to diagnose FTD. For these reasons, perhaps, and because of the rhetorical impact on readers of bizarre transgressions, the literature on FTD tends to highlight egregious acts. And some of the behaviors of some FTD patients are sociopathic. In one series of 12 FTD patients with predominantly right-side disease, extensive interviews with patients and families uncovered 7 with some criminal behavior, 10 with aggression, 2 who had committed some sort of financial recklessness, and 5 with reported sexually deviant behavior (Mychack *et al.* 2001; the authors do not define the criteria for these non-exclusive categories). In another series of 16 patients with FTD, 4 had committed sexual or touching violations, 3 had violated major traffic laws, 2 had committed physical assaults, 2 had committed other crimes, and 2 had urinated or exposed themselves in public (Mendez, Chen, *et al.* 2005; see Mendez, 2006 for an overview of transgressions reported in the literature). FTD patients also resemble sociopaths and some frontal lesion patients in not showing remorse or guilt about transgressions they commit.

Nevertheless, it is clear that in general, FTD patients tend to be much less aggressive or violent than sociopaths or some frontal lesion patients, and unlike sociopaths they rarely exploit people through cons or elaborate deceptions. So far as we know, none of the FTD patients we ourselves have studied to date has committed a crime or injured anyone, so we have not been able to assess their experience of guilt or remorse, or the absence of such emotions. But we certainly have not observed apologies or expressions of regret for the myriad small transgressions they commit or their failures to respond to family members in need.

For the most part, however, our research so far suggests that the phenomenology of FTD is not fraught with high drama. Rather, the patient's relationships die by a thousand cuts. As the disease appears and advances, interactions become awkward and the afflicted person commits myriad small offenses, inflicts innumerable small social injuries, and gradually ceases to show concern or offer help. The afflicted person slowly becomes less inhibited and more preoccupied with selfish desires, or else becomes lazy and indifferent. For a while, these changes can be perceived as among the vicissitudes of normal personality and relationships. Family members may generally attribute the afflicted person's changing behavior to a life-stage or to the dissolution of the person's love for their spouse and children. Family members may even initially suppose that they themselves are at fault, wondering if they are unlovable.

It seems that the decision to seek clinical help is often precipitated by one or more particularly egregious transgressions that cannot readily be explained away. Dramatically bizarre breaches may be infrequent, however, and are probably uncommon in the first year or two of the development of the disease. It is not known, and not easy to discover, how many people are afflicted with FTD without ever being brought to a clinic, and how many are taken to see a physician but are never correctly diagnosed. What is clear, however, is that most cases that are eventually diagnosed have shown mundane signs of FTD for years beforehand. So there is a pressing need to characterize just what distinguishes everyday FTD from normal behavior and from other disorders. If and when treatments are developed that can arrest or even reverse the progression of the disease, it will be vitally important to identify FTD in its early stages, before there is extensive or irreversible damage to the patient's neurological and social relational systems. In the meanwhile, it is still a great relief to most family members and friends to discover that the deterioration of their relationship with the afflicted person has an organic cause: somehow it is consoling to know that the problem is fundamentally neurological, not purely relational.

Family members report changes in the patient's personality, but their informal and necessarily tendentious descriptions cannot accurately capture the precise details and contingencies of daily interaction. Their reports are unsystematic, based on imperfect recall of events, and biased by the family's objectives in bringing the patient to the clinic, often despite the patient's resistance. Moreover, it is important to note that FTD consists of insidious, gradual *changes* in social relational behavior, emotions, and motives: a lazy person who has always been lazy does not have FTD, he's just a bum. A selfish, insensitive person who has always been obnoxious does not have FTD, he is simply a jerk. So longitudinal data would be invaluable, and we have begun to collect this. Ideally, one would like to compare participant observation and recordings of social interactions in natural settings *before* the onset of FTD with the same types of data collected at various stages of the disease's progression. But this is not often feasible. Conversation analysis in conjunction with participant observation reveal potentially diagnostic social relational aberrations that probably emerge years before the patient commits any horrific violations—if they ever do. We need to build on these insights to develop sensitive diagnostic tools.

## Social Motives Fade Away While Other Motives Remain Intact

We already know that the patterns of interaction described in this volume do not exhaust the distinctive features of the everyday social lives of our subjects Romeo, Steve, Kelly, Juno, Louise, Vera, and Ned; analysis of our corpus of recordings and field notes is on-going. We do not yet know how representative our sample of seven patients is, so we look forward to working with additional patients and discovering additional distinguishing characteristics of the social relationships of FTD patients. However, the conversation analyses and participant observation of the members of the Social Relations in FTD Project whose chapters appear in this volume already show that FTD patients sometimes do not initiate new topics, do not ask personal or other questions, and give minimal answers or answers that repeat a question phrase. They may interrupt or switch the topic to themselves. FTD patients sometimes provide insufficient or excessive information when identifying others. FTD patients sometimes initiate conversations with strangers or, conversely, abruptly leave interactions when it is socially awkward to do so. They sometimes ignore obvious suffering and do not come to the aid of persons who have a salient need or problem. They may fail to fulfill requests, even when it is easy or important to do so. They rarely take offense or express resentment, and they placidly do things that embarrass others without any indication that they feel any embarrassment themselves.

Understanding of FTD must build on such descriptions of its natural social behavioral phenomenology—FTD *is* a disease of social relationships. But to understand FTD we need to go beneath the behavioral phenomenology to make inferences about causal mechanisms at the level of emotions and motives, and beyond. This is especially crucial for the project of linking the social relational psychology of FTD to its neuropathology and etiology. We need to understand the socio-emotional, relational-motivational phenotype of FTD in order to discern *how* the breakdown of neural systems results in the breakdown in social relationships—and to discover how those neural systems normally function to sustain functional, meaningful, satisfying relationships.

What *is* going wrong in FTD? An extensive body of theory and research shows that normal social relationships in all contexts in all cultures are organized by four fundamental relational models, Communal Sharing, Authority Ranking, Equality Matching, and Market Pricing (Fiske 1991; Haslam 2004a; Fiske and Haslam 2005). Everyday sociality depends on intrinsic motivations to seek, to form, to sustain and to repair these four basic forms of relationship (Fiske 2002). That is, people depend on moral emotions to regulate their own and others' behavior to conform to each of these relational models. So it is natural to hypothesize that FTD patients' social relational dysfunctionality may result from diminution of the social motives and moral emotions necessary to functional, meaningful, satisfying relationships of some or all of these four fundamental types of relationships. And indeed our participant observation and conversation analysis tentatively suggest that FTD patients lack the affiliative social motivation to be "with" other people in Communal Sharing relationships, along with the moral emotions crucial for Communal Sharing: embarrassment, shame, concern for others, compassion, empathy, and love. The patients we have studied also seem to lack the Authority Ranking motivation to sustain status, as well as the emotions related to taking offense at being disrespected or belittled: they appear to have little or no pride and they usually don't get angry when bossed around.

When our subject Steve displays total disregard for taking turns or following rules playing pool, and lacks embarrassment about ignoring the rules, this suggests that he, at least, also lacks the motivation for evenly balanced Equality Matching or the moral emotions that would regulate his turn-taking; further investigations will determine whether deficits in motivation for equality and emotional concern about even-matching (such as envy) are characteristic of other patients. The patients we observed and interacted with also appear unconcerned about their finances and unmotivated to economize. For Steve, the first sign that his wife, Anne, noticed of the change that turned out to be FTD was that Steve bought her gifts, including expensive jewelry; this was unlike him—he had rarely shopped for anything before this. Ned stops going to work, and Kelly does not seem to worry about the consequences of ceasing her lessons. On two occasions Vera tried to give Michael, her ethnographer, over \$100 in cash, and she likes to buy people meals and tip waiters; apparently she has enough money that this is not a problem. Despite their apparently precarious finances, Romeo wastes money on frivolous purchases and is totally unconcerned about their loss of health insurance. This suggests a probable deficit in Market Pricing motivations. Perhaps, then, FTD patients lose motivations and emotions required to seek, create, sustain, repair, and regulate all four fundamental types of social relationships. Moreover, the limited evidence suggests that perhaps patients lose Market Pricing motivation before they lose all of the Communal Sharing motivation. These results in natural settings greatly extend tests performed in the clinic of deficiencies in several related emotions (Mendez, Anderson and Shapira 2005; Passant *et al.* 2005; Snowden *et al.* 2001; see also Beer *et al.* 2003).

In sum, we need much more data, but at this point the CA and participant observation with the first seven patients strongly suggest that they are deficient in Communal Sharing emotions and motives of shame, embarrassment, affection, affiliativeness, empathy, or compassion. There is also clear evidence for a lack of Authority Ranking emotions and motives such as pride, and anger when demeaned or diminished. Market Pricing emotions and motives also appear to be deficient, but there is insufficient evidence to draw conclusions, and we still know little about Equality Matching emotions and motives.

People typically have a variety of motives for cooperative sociality. People do their duty and discharge their responsibilities because they genuinely care about others, but also because they are sensitive to norms and social expectations, because they care about their reputation, or because they seek the social status that comes with achievement. The sociomoral emotions and motives that bolster 'responsibility' vary from person to person and from one responsibility to another. People are responsible about performance in some areas out of deferential respect for—or fear of—authority, or from a pastoral, 'paternalistic' sense of responsibility for subordinates. People are often motivated by their identification with their family, team, work group, or organization: they want the camaraderie of membership, they want the prestige of notable contributions, and they want the group to prosper. What is striking about FTD is that *all* of these social motives appear to wane together, leaving only the basic non-relational motives that humans share with mammalian species that are asocial: hunger, sexual appetite, fear, curiosity.

Which is to say that FTD patients do not lose all motives or emotions. They are still hungry, and still interested in sex (Mendez and Cummings 2003; Zald and Kim 2001; Rule *et al.* 2002). After the onset of his FTD symptoms, Ned's interest in pornography became, if anything, more overt, upsetting his wife considerably (Fiske, Sept.10, 2008: field notes). When Ned's caretakers fail to have his dinner ready when he expects it at promptly at 6:00, he gets "really agitated," Fred reports. Indeed, Ned gained a lot of weight after he developed FTD. Another FTD patient was pulled over for speeding in his hurry to get an ice-cream cone (Mendez, personal communication). Fred says that Ned is an avid participant in table games and continues to enjoy attending college basketball games. Some FTD patients express uninhibited curiosity about interesting objects, reflected in their "utilization behavior" (the unrestrained exploration of novel or intriguing objects). Another indication of curiosity is Louise's interrupting her daughter to ask Michael, "Are you trying to grow a beard?" (Smith, Sept. 24, 2003a: field notes). Vera asks Michael a series of personal questions on more than one occasion (Smith, Chapter 3, this volume; videos Nov. 23, 2003a and Dec. 11, 2003d). After I asked Ned about his family, he asked me if I had any grandchildren (Fiske, Sept. 10, 2008: field notes). FTD patients also startle, as Kelly does when the glasses of water spill (Torrisi, Feb. 23, 2007: field notes), and Smith observed Vera utter a dismayed emphasized in-breath with raised eye-brows, open mouth, and raised pull-back (Smith, Chapter 3, this volume; video Dec. 11, 2003D). They evidently experience fear: FTD patients do not commonly walk in traffic, burn themselves on stoves, or disregard their personal safety in other ways.

When they are not getting what they want or are having difficulties performing a task, Ned, Steve, and Romeo make noises or gestures that suggest frustration. Both Romeo and Steve often grunt, apparently with effortful frustration, when they are doing tasks they have been assigned—usually self-maintenance tasks such as getting shoes on, putting fruit on their cereal, or Romeo's putting photographs of his recent first communion into an album (Mates, Oct. 22, 2006; Nov. 28, 2006: field notes respectively). It is difficult to determine whether by their grunts they intend to convey annoyance at being told to perform these tasks, or whether these noises are non-communicative reflections of frustration with the tasks themselves. We do not know if they make these sounds when they are alone. Although Romeo is usually passively compliant, he expresses apparent frustration if he is told to do something that interferes with another activity he is presently engaged in.

Ned's agitation when dinner does not arrive promptly suggests that he experiences frustration. Vera's daughter, Linda, says that Vera gets angry when the diagnosis of FTD is mentioned, insisting that the problem is only with her memory, and she repeatedly buys gingko biloba, which she hopes will alleviate her memory problem (Smith Nov. 11, 2003: field notes; video Dec. 11, 2003). When Louise's daughter Dana says that Dr. Mendez "took one look at Louise" and immediately diagnosed FTD, Louise replies with indignation "not <u>one</u> look. I didn't look at him and go 'eughhhh'," putting her hands to side of her head, her thumbs to her ears, and wiggling her fingers (Smith, Sept. 3, 2003: field notes). This could indicate that Louise still experiences some residual embarrassment, but the childish gestures suggest frustration, and that she lacks embarrassment and is, instead, simply irritated that Dana's characterization of the event is inconsistent with her own memory of the events. Vera habitually insists on paying for meals at restaurants, and she shows indignation when Michael tries to slip some money to her daughter, Susan, for his share of lunch (Smith, Nov. 11, 2003: field notes). These everyday expressions of appetites for food and sex, of curiosity, surprise, and frustration, show that FTD patients do not lose all emotions or motives: non-social emotions and motives seem more or less intact.

In short, we theorize, and our observations tentatively confirm, that FTD patients specifically lose the emotions and motives that are necessary to social relationships. As a result, they fail to do what they need to do to sustain their social relationships over the long-term, so their relationships deteriorate on the job, in the family, and in recreational and civic settings. For quite a while, however, they continue to be able to respond fairly well to the *immediate moment* of the interaction: they listen; they may notice, recognize, and sometimes respond to others' non-verbal emotional signals; they reply; and they comply. But this immediate social reactivity slowly fades away—and even before it fades, FTD patients' relationships deteriorate because social relationships demand more than moment to moment responses—relationships only function when people are motivated to be sociable, and are only rewarding and trusting when people are emotionally committed (Fiske 2002).

In this volume, Torrisi, Mates, Joaquin, and others discuss the right ventral medial prefrontal and anterior temporal cortical areas whose degeneration is associated with these deficits in social motives and moral emotions. It is also possible to speculatively connect these relational motives and moral emotions with emerging knowledge in social neurochemistry. Oxytocin (OT) appears to play an especially pivotal role in maternal behavior and also in female pair bonding in "monogamous" species of mammals, where a closely related neuropeptide, arginine vasopressin (AVP), appears to mediate pair bonding in males (Uvnäs-Moberg 1998; Carter *et al.* 1999; Kendrick 2000; Young *et al.* 2001; Insel and Young 2001, de Bono 2003). In human mothers, delivering a baby, skin-contact with the baby, the infant's massaging of the breast, and nursing all release oxytocin from the posterior pituitary, mediated by the paraventricular nucleus of the hypothalamus (Panksepp 1998, 246–260; Matthiesen *et al.* 2001). It seems likely that OT mediates human affiliation in other relations, as well (Fiske 2004). One possibility is that the appetitive phase of affiliative bonding is mediated by the activity of the ventral tegmental area dopamine–nucleus accumbens shell pathway, while the consumatory phase is independently mediated by the central corticolimbic projections of the u-opiate system of the medial basal arcuate nucleus (Depue and Morrone-Strupinsky 2005). Plasma OT levels are correlated with how close one feels to one's partner (Grewen *et al.* 2005).

A core deficit of FTD is patients' apparent loss of the consumatory feelings of love or "closeness"—that is, deficits in the motives and emotions that support Communal Sharing relationships. So it is plausible to suppose that FTD involves decreased production of OT and AVP, loss of receptors for OT and AVP, or damage to the neural systems that respond to these affectional peptides. Little is known about whether or how OT and AVP are related to social motives and moral emotions of other relationships. The only clearly relevant literature is on the role of serotonin in depression and anxiety disorders. Depression often involves feelings of guilt or worthlessness, and is linked to loss, sadness, and social withdrawal. Some anxiety disorders involve social relational concerns such as the preoccupation of some OCD patients with the possibility that they may have harmed someone or violated some social norm. So FTD may involve disruptions of some of the brain's many serotonin pathways. Dopamine systems in the ventral tegmental area are also likely to be involved via their extensive innervations from the ventral medial prefrontal cortex (see Mates, Chapter 6, this volume). So the most likely cause of some of the deficits in Communal Sharing motives and emotions is the interruption of pathways connecting the right orbitofrontal and anterior temporal cortices with emotional and motivational systems mediated by OT, AVP, serotonin, and dopamine.

## Multiple Methods for Investigating Social Motives and Moral Emotions in Ftd

Conversation analysis provides a very detailed, precise description of interactions, a description that goes beyond what an interlocutor or observer could describe without this kind of meticulous study of recordings. The CA of the contributors to this volume demonstrates that the social interactions of FTD patients are unusual in several respects. Traditional CA stops at description, refraining from attributing psychological states, and few CA researchers make quantitative comparisons across situations or persons. However, I hope this chapter demonstrates that CA provides a wonderful foundation for making inferences about psychological states and traits, including quantitative comparisons.

In the Social Relations in FTD Project (SRFTDP) we use CA in conjunction with several other methods that are complementary and synergistic. In the background behind the CA in this volume is the participant observation ethnography of the authors who interacted with patients and their families as normally as possible. Trying to carry on normal interactions and form relationships with the patients, the ethnographers themselves experienced frustration, irritation, disgust, hurt feelings, boredom, confusion, surprise, and sometimes warm affection. That is, the ethnographers experienced firsthand what it is like to try to relate to FTD patients, and then recorded these experiences, including their emotional reactions and attributions, in their field notes. This provides a more immediate, detailed, precise, reliable, and in some respects more complete record of the "natural history" of FTD. This is the essence of participant observation (PO): using oneself as the instrument of observation, participating while translating the experience into field notes that form the basis for description, interpretation, and analysis. What is unique about the SRFTDP is that we can go back and forth between the field notes and the CA. We can use the CA to understand precisely what actions and patterns are evoking specific emotional reactions and attributions in the participant observer. Conversely, we can use the participants' experiences, recorded in their field notes and discussed in our lab meetings, to understand the consequences and sequelae of acts and patterns that CA picks up. Without CA, the participant observer doesn't see precisely what s/he is reacting to; without PO, the conversation analyst doesn't know the psycho-social consequences of the conversational breaches.

A third dimension of the SRFTDP is to compare the CA and PO with family reports (FR) about the patient, permitting us to understand how the participant observers' experiences resemble and differ from the experience of family members whose relationships extend back before the onset of the disorder, who interact much more frequently with the patient over a wider range of situations, and who have far more at stake. Then we can compare CA, PO, and FR with the neurologist's and nurse's clinical impressions (CI). The CI differ from the other data because the clinicians have far, far more experience with and expertise about FTD and other disorders than anyone else, but on the other hand their interactions with the patient and family are highly structured and atypical of everyday life. We are videotaping clinical interviews to determine precisely how patients' interactions with the neurologist resemble and differ from the same patients interactions in everyday life.

CA, PO, FR, and CI are all qualitative data, rich and valid. But they have the limitations of qualitative data: they are difficult to replicate, they are uncontrolled, and comparisons with other populations cannot be statistically tested. So we are applying behavior sampling (BS) methods to measure rates of occurrence of key behaviors. These analyses use both focal-following and time-sampling protocols, and will yield rates per unit time, rates per word, and rates using various conversational context denominators. As the examples briefly cited in this chapter illustrate, FTD patients' rates of various conversational acts and omissions differ dramatically and significantly from normal controls' rates of the same behaviors. We then plan to use the BS data to construct an 'ethogram' of the social behaviors that are characteristic of FTD and distinguish it from normal behavior and other pathologies.

Like the results from the qualitative methods, BS yields ecologically valid data about the behavior that defines and constitutes FTD: dysfunctional social relations. It has the merit of enabling quantitative comparison that controls for various denominators such as time, utterances, words, questions, topics, or whatever may be of interest. But the naturalistic validity of CA, PO, FR, CI, and BS necessarily means that there are no controls and limited comparability regarding the age, gender, education, personality, roles, or number of their interlocutors, or the social or physical context. The lack of constancy of these factors that certainly influence social interaction limits the inferences that can be drawn from the data. So we are using two other methods that control the setting and stimuli, although they consequently have less ecological validity. First, we have developed behavioral tests (BT) of social motives and moral emotions in standardized but naturalistic situations, using the methods of experimental social psychology. Each of these tests is designed to correspond to typical FTD behaviors reported in clinical reports of FTD and observed by us in our fieldwork. Most of the tests are also adaptations of classical, well-replicated social psychology experiments. For example, a test that has been used successfully with frontal lesion patients is to ask them to give an example of a situation in which they experienced embarrassment; frontal lesion patients reveal more intimate, humiliating experiences than controls, apparently because they don't feel as embarrassed to tell them (Beer *et al.* 2003). To provide another convergent window onto patients' experience of moral and non-moral emotions, we are also using physiological measurements (PM), including skin conductance, blood pressure, and heart rate, in response to social and non-social situations. The situations we present are based on clinical reports of FTD, FR, and our own PO and BS.

We use CA, PO, FR, CI, BS, BT, and PM in conjunction with results from psychological and neurological tests (NT), and of course structural and functional neuroimaging (NI). Eventually we also plan to use autopsy reports (AR) to correlate with these data. Each of these ten types of data complements the others, providing convergent evidence about the phenomenology, mechanisms, and causes of FTD, and at the same time validating (or invalidating) each of the other methods. Measurement of our constructs, such as embarrassment or compassion, or of any constructs, requires the use of multiple measures of each construct (Campbell and D.W. Fiske 1959; D.W. Fiske 1982). All measurements are determined by multiple factors, including many that are extraneous to the construct they aim to measure. So if we measure constructs using only one method, it is impossible to determine what contributes to the measurements; correlations among measures based on the same method may result (indeed, often do result) largely or entirely from method effects, rather than from true associations among the constructs themselves. Hence the measures used must have maximally distinct sources of error and bias. To assess the validity of any construct, we must measure it using multiple methods and examine the associations of each of those measures with multiple measures of other constructs, some of which our theory tells us should be associated with the key construct and some of which should be independent of it. Only when we examine this multi-method, multi-trait matrix can we assess the validity of the constructs or the methods. Without this strategy it is impossible to know what, if anything, we are actually measuring (Campbell and D.W. Fiske 1959, D.W. Fiske, 1982). The SRFTDP aims to meet this criterion for convergent and discriminant validity. Combining CA, PO, FR, CI, BS, BT, PM, NT, NI, and AR on the same patients and controls, we hope that eventually we will be able to determine the nature of meaningful social relationships and the specific neurochemical processes and neuroanatomical systems that are necessary to sustain them.

## Why Dispassionate Rationality is Insufficient to Sustain Relationships

We have far to go and many challenges to meet to fully implement this research plan, but in the final section of this chapter let us return to the question of why FTD patients fail to sustain social relationships that are meaningful and satisfying to their associates and families. In the first years of FTD, patients' memory and reasoning are typically more or less normal and they are aware of what is going on around them. Their perceptual and motor processes function well. For example, Steve was a composer and Kelly was a professional piano teacher; both continued to be extremely proficient piano players even when their disease had progressed considerably, and Steve could still sing well. They seem to understand the personalities of their family members, friends and associates. Generally they are fully aware of other people's mental states, and sometimes they respond to non-verbal facial and postural cues of emotions. The sociocultural knowledge patients have acquired over four or five decades is accessible to them: they know what they should do according to general norms and specific role obligations. They are aware of the probable consequences of their actions. Why isn't this sufficient?

Our theory is that the core and defining deficit of FTD patients is a loss of social motives and moral emotions. Yet they retain basic non-social drives, including motives and emotions such as far of physical harm and pain, startle response, curiosity, hunger, thirst, and sexual desire. In the early stages afflicted persons may retain near normal memory, knowledge of social norms, and social reasoning abilities: they typically understand the consequences of their choices. In short, they are the dispassionate rational actors that are the agents who constitute the core of most theory in economics, behaviorism, and evolutionary psychology. But we think that FTD patients demonstrate that there is much more to intrinsically rewarding, mutually meaningful social relationships: participants must care about their partners and about the relationships as ends in themselves.

The dominant theory of human behavior is that people act rationally to maximize their utility. Social scientists recognize that rationality is constrained by information costs and operationalized through heuristics, and that people are not fully aware of all of their motives or "automatic" cognitive processes. Rational actor theory acknowledges that a person's utility calculations take internalized norms into account, as well as potential social sanctions. Allowing for these factors, rational actor theory posits that human action is driven by dispassionate reasoning about the optimal means to achieve ends. FTD patients in the early stages of their affliction are rational actors, yet their social relationships disintegrate. Why is dispassionate rationality insufficient to sustain enduring, satisfying relationships? To answer this question, let us consider the nature of dispassionate human rationality.

### *Failure to appreciate the consequences*

Rational action requires knowledge of the consequences of action. Yet if people rely on the feedback of their personal experience to guide their social behavior, they will systematically and seriously underestimate the consequences of their own social failings, misdemeanors, and transgressions. When I was a child, my mother told me that that if I were mean to my playmates or rude to their parents, I would not get invited back to play again. But, my mother said, your friends and their parents won't ever *tell* you why they haven't invited you back—or even mention that they are not inviting you. You just won't hear from them again. My mother's dictum captures an important general principle about social relationships. When you commit an offense, people tend to conceal the fact that they feel hurt or offended, wishing to avoid a confrontational "scene." Furthermore, people like to gossip, and the most appealing gossip concerns social judgments and especially stories of transgressions. Yet such gossip is often invisible to the person whose actions are evaluated. People you offend may retaliate in ways that cause you trouble, without your ever discovering that they did so. By stabbing you in the back covertly, vengeful people protect themselves from your retaliation. The lesson is that people who are offended often avoid confronting the miscreant, preferring to sanction misbehavior by withdrawal, indirect recriminations, or covert revenge. This means that many important consequences of social misaction are difficult or impossible for the actor to discern.

The consequences of malfeasance extend beyond the victim's retaliation or withdrawal from the relationship. If you offend someone, they may tell others. If you cheat them, they are nearly certain to complain to their friends, who in turn are likely to enjoy gossiping about it. If you steal a tool from someone who tells 10 people, who each tell 10 others, who each tell 10 others, who in turn tell 10 others, then 11,111 people hear about your wrongdoing (1 + 10 + 100 + 1000 + 10,000, assuming no overlap in reporting). Thus gossip may quickly spread throughout the entire community—the thief's total network of potential associates. Each person who hears of the theft becomes distrustful and avoids forming potentially beneficial relationships with the thief, at an enormous cost that the thief is unlikely to have fully anticipated. People probably don't think about the geometric spread of reputations though gossip, and if they don't, they will underestimate the ramifications of wrong-doing.

Some sanctions come too late to repair a relationship. A student caught cheating may be expelled and an employee caught embezzling may be fired. A person caught in adultery may be divorced or murdered, while a disloyal gang member may be expelled or executed.

What this all means—what my mother was telling me—is that people cannot easily *learn* to be good based on their own personal experience. The most serious consequences of misbehavior are often invisible, unforeseeable, and irreversible. To get along with each other, people have to be motivated by something more than what they can see of the consequences of their own behavior. While FTD patients in the early stages can often still perceive others' reactions to their acts, this is not sufficient, because most of the most serious ultimate consequences are invisible.

Still, despite this maternal wisdom, it might seem that a reflective person could ultimately figure out the importance of good social behavior. But would intelligent observation and analysis of events lead a wise person to be good? In everyday life, people are often faced with temptations to violate social relationships: a person has to choose between satisfying a hedonistic impulse and doing the right thing. A researcher has to decide whether to check the data entry, or just hope it was done right; who will ever find out? A forager who kills a small animal asks himself, shall I just eat it here in the bush without telling anyone, or bring it back to share with the whole band? People are sometimes tempted to have extra-marital affairs; do they choose the immediate gratification or their marital commitment? What would we expect people to do if they make a dispassionate choice between such alternatives?

In individualist cultures, at least, people's expectations of personal success often far exceed the objective probabilities (Langer 1975). This illusion of control is especially strong when people make a carefully considered choice, are familiar with the stimulus or response choices, are involved in the situation, and perceive the situation as a competition against one or more other persons. Of course, this perfectly describes the situation of a person deciding whether they can get away with a social transgression. People believe that they are more skillful than average and less likely than average to be harmed or to suffer an early death; people also over generalize from their experience of successfully evading low probability risks (Slovic *et al.* 1982). Weinstein (1989) has repeatedly shown that Americans are unrealistically optimistic about their lack of susceptibility to health risks and other hazards, especially when they extrapolate from their own past experience.

In fact, people are unrealistically optimistic about their expectations in every domain (Armor and Taylor 2002). Armor and Taylor (2002, 334) write, "One of the most robust findings in the psychology of prediction is that people's predictions tend to be optimistically biased. By a number of metrics and across a variety of domains, people have been found to assign higher probabilities to their attainment of desirable outcomes than either objective criteria or logical analysis warrants." This optimistic bias resists disconfirmation and experimental manipulations intended to reduce it. It operates in predictions of social events (Dunning *et al.* 1990). Thus if a person afflicted with FTD reflects about whether they can get away with violating social norms, they will often erroneously conclude that they are likely to succeed.

The more distant the consequences and the more times a person has avoided unfortunate consequences of an action, the greater the bias in over-estimating success and invulnerability. People may not take the trouble to put on seat belts, thinking "I have been driving for years and never had an accident." Even if a person initially fears detection, if they once do commit a transgression and get away with it, their anxiety is likely to diminish. Extrapolating from successful past evasions, they will become progressively more cocksure as they go along. As a teenager, I remember my friends reassuring me as we were sneaking into a closed gym to play basketball: "Come on! We've done this lots of times before. What are you worried about?" (We got caught.)

Moreover, the more people want something, the more they are inclined to believe they are likely to get it. Human reasoning is partial; what people *want* affects their analyses of what is *likely* (Kunda 1990, 1999). "People are more likely to arrive at conclusions they want to arrive at" (Kunda 1990, 480), evidently because they work harder to access information in memory consistent with their desires, search harder for desired features of situations, and are prone to select decision heuristics that guide them toward their wishes. Furthermore, the greater the benefit of something, the lower the perceived risk of the hazards it entails (Fishoff *et al.* 1978). This correlation seems to be mediated by the affect associated with activities and events: when people like something, they judge its risks to be much lower than when they dislike something (Slovic *et al.* 1999). Faced with a temptation to do something she wants to do, or to shirk a responsibility, a dispassionately reasoning FTD patient will tend to conclude that it is OK to do it and that in any case the risks are minimal—even when the objective expected utility is negative. Since a person afflicted with FTD still has basic selfish drives for food, sex, safety, and comfort, they are likely to pursue these needs when they underestimate the likelihood of sanctions.

### Misjudgments of small and compound probabilities

When estimating probabilities people consistently ignore base rates (Tversky and Kahneman 1982). Applied to temptation and self-control, this suggests that even if people are aware of the base rate of detection of transgression in the community as a whole, they will ignore that information when estimating their own chances of getting away with cheating. People will be prone to believe that *they* can get away with doing what they want to do without getting caught.

Moreover, when the probability of an event is small, people act as if the probability is zero, even if they know better (Kahneman and Tversky 1979). This decision heuristic can get FTD patients (and others) into a lot of trouble if they are making a decision about a defection or transgression for which the penalty is substantial. If the chances of being caught are small and people act as if the effective probability is zero, they will give in to temptation no matter how great the cost of being sanctioned if they are caught. The expected cost is the product of the probability of being caught and the penalty if caught; if they act as if there is *no* chance of being caught, people will treat the expected cost as zero, regardless of the magnitude of the penalty.

Furthermore, in most such situations, what matters is whether you *ever* get caught. If you are shoplifting, committing adultery, cheating, or embezzling, being detected once may cost you far more than you gained from all the transgressions put together. If the probability of detection in each instance is independent, then the chance of always getting away with it is a compound probability, $p^n$: the chance of getting away with it each time, $p$, to an exponent which is the number of transgressions. Human reasoning errors become quite egregious when dealing with compound events: People overestimate the probabilities of conjunctive events (the odds of something occurring every time) and underestimate the probabilities of disjunctive events (the odds that something will happen at least once; Cohen and Hansel 1958; Bar-Hillel 1973; Tversky and Kahneman 1983). People prefer compound gambles in which their odds of success are favorable at each step: "the probabilities of the individual stages in a chain of events thus appear to have greater influence on the evaluation of the whole chain's probability than the number of stages in question" (Bar-Hillel 1973, 405).

This bias is quite pronounced when people think about their own exploits: people vastly overestimate their compound probability of being successful every time. In one experiment, subjects in every experimental condition overestimated their chances of correctly guessing *all* of a series of locations of a hidden ticket; their overestimation of success on all guesses increased exponentially with the number of locations they were to guess (Cohen *et al.* 1982). When the true odds were $2^{-24}$ (about 0.00000006), subjects guessed that their odds of making all guesses correctly were 1 in 20. That is, subjects were over-estimating their chances of success by a factor of 833,333. Subjects' overestimates are a function of a power of the number of alternatives they are guessing among at each stage, and increase exponentially with the number of stages (guesses they have to make). That is, the distortion increases extremely rapidly with increasing complexity of events and increasing number of events. In an important series of studies of reasoning about other matters, Gigerenzer and his colleagues (e.g., Gigerenzer and Hertwig 1999) have shown that Bayesian reasoning improves where problems are represented in terms of frequencies rather than probabilities: overestimations of conjoint probabilities (and, in one study, illusions of control) are reduced substantially. We do not know just how people reason about social defections. But even when reasoning with frequencies, people still considerably overestimate conjoint probabilities.

If we can extrapolate at all from this extensive body of research to everyday social life, the implication is clear: people are not going to understand how likely they are to get caught. If any of the biases in reasoning about compound probabilities—let alone all of them—operate in everyday life, people will hugely overestimate their chances of getting away with social transgressions. Suppose there is a .99 probability of getting away with the theft of food from a communal store, and suppose that a hungry person steals every day. If the chances of detection of each transgression are independent, the probability of escaping punishment for a year is .026. After two years, the probability of always getting away with it is below .0007. Of course, the crucial assumption, that the probabilities of detection on each occasion are independent, is not entirely valid. But there are innumerable chance factors affecting detection of defection, and together, these chance factors may generally be independent in the long run. The conclusion is clear: Dispassionate reasoners don't understand compound probabilities, so they are likely to be vastly overconfident that they will never get caught. FTD patients are dispassionate reasoners, so when they choose between right and wrong, although they know the consequences of getting caught, they will be overconfident that they will get away with what they want to do.

Two other, related properties of human psychology lead people into social problems. The first I call egocentric oblivion. I stay at work late for what seem to me perfectly good reasons, not foreseeing the disruption in family plans. Perhaps I forgot, or never knew, that my wife was making a soufflé and had committed herself to go to a meeting right after dinner. Or I'm at a party and I tell a very long, exciting (I think) story about an African adventure. I love the story, but others are bored, and irritated that I'm monopolizing the conversation. In general, people often fail to anticipate that their actions will offend someone and may not even recognize afterwards that they have done so. A person cannot know, or reliably attend to, everything in another person's life or mind, which leads to unintended slights and unrecognized oversights. It's impossible to see the world through another person's eyes. That's egocentric oblivion.

The second untoward psychological property I call empathic discounting. I can understand that my son doesn't like my telling him how to wash dishes; I probably didn't like it when my father told me how to wash dishes, either. But sometimes I fail to appreciate that my son could be just as irritated by what I do as I am when others do the same thing to me. In general, people cannot adequately feel the depth of others' feelings. I know that the authors of the manuscript I am reviewing will be annoyed at many of my critiques, but I don't really realize that they will be as irate as I am when they review *my* manuscripts. I know they won't like to hear the criticisms but, since my suggestions are certainly valid, I don't expect them to be angry. In any case, I can't *feel* their aggravation as fully as I feel my own in the same circumstances. So in my actions I discount other people's feelings relative to my own. Under some circumstances, the result of discounted empathy may be friction, discord, and perhaps endless rounds of retaliation.

Although we are all capable of perceiving expressed emotions and reading other minds, this isn't sufficient to sustain good relationships because it is nearly impossible to fully take the perspectives of our partners, let alone mere associates. Like everyone else, FTD patients surely are vulnerable to egocentric obliviousness and empathic discounting.

### *Hyperbolic discounting: The value of a reward or punishment is inversely proportional to how far in the future it is*

Probably the single biggest obstacle to sustaining long-term social relationships is not a limitation of reasoning as such, but the temporal structure of motivation. Immediate rewards are exceedingly tantalizing and immediate punishments look frightfully painful, while remote rewards and punishments are negligible incentives. Even without all the biases of human reasoning, this would probably make rationally reasoning people succumb to most temptations to cheat or defect. Humans, like all animals, discount the value of future rewards and punishments approximately in inverse proportion to their (expected) distance in the future (for reviews see Frank 1988; Ainslie and Haslam 1992; and Gallistel and Gibbon 2000). This is called hyperbolic discounting. This hyperbolic temporal discounting is ubiquitous and consistent among humans and other animals for subjectively certain outcomes, not just uncertain ones. All dog trainers know this; you must reward or punish *immediately*—it's no use doing it a minute or two later.

Hyperbolic discounting often results in temporal inconsistencies in preferences. If a person (or any animal) is choosing between a small reward and a big one that are both far in the future, of course the big reward outweighs the small one. However, if the small reward is available right now and the big one is fairly far in the future, people choose the current reward over the much larger but much more distant one.[2] We see this in risky sexual behavior where the immediate pleasure often outweighs the small probability of contracting debilitating or even deadly diseases whose consequences are far in the future. We experience this when we succumb to immediate temptation to eat delicious foods that result in obesity and ill-health far in the future.

Even otherwise fully rational dispassionate actors cannot resist the lure of immediate pleasures because they are hyperbolically discounting the future; they cannot exert the self control needed to make arduous exertions or painful sacrifices. The ultimate future costs have little subjective weight. In functional or subjective value terms, the result of hyperbolic discounting is that present action is prone to be inconsistent with long-term preferences and overall utilities. In evolutionary terms, this means that unless countervailing mechanisms are operating, organisms will generally fail to realize major long-term adaptive needs that are inconsistent with short-term motives. For many organisms this may not usually be a major problem because they have few important long-term adaptive strategies that cannot be achieved by continually pursuing immediate appetites. And if expected survival is short, there will be few temporal inconsistencies in adaptive 'preference' mechanisms. But human survival and well-being depend on long-term social coordination, cooperation, exchange, trust, and loyalty. In human social life, current basic pleasures often incur social penalties in the future; and current efforts or costs

---

2.   A perfectly rational economic actor might discount exponentially, which would result in consistent choices because exponential curves do not cross. But hyperbolic discounting curves often do cross, so that what the actor wants when one reward or punishment is immediate and the other is distant is not what the actor wants when both are more distant.

have social rewards only later, after considerable delays. Very often, the basic animal drives for food, sex, safety, comfort, and exploration are elicited by opportunities for immediate satisfaction, while the benefits of social relationships are deferred. This is as true of FTD patients as anyone else.

### Non-linearity and asymmetry of losses and gains

A rational person would value outcomes according to their expected value: the product of the utility times the probability of the event. However, when humans make decisions, they subjectively overvalue certain outcomes and undervalue others compared to their expected value and, indeed, compared to a linear function of the quantity of money or goods. Prospect theory, which is supported by a huge body of data, characterizes how people value certain or risky gains and losses (Kahneman and Tversky 1979; Tversky and Kahneman 1991). First, prospect theory posits that people are more concerned about losses than gains—they are loss averse. For example, few people will accept an even chance of winning $105 or paying $100. This is formally described as a utility function that is steeper for losses than for gains. Second, people are often willing to take risks when seeking large gains, but people prefer a certain small loss to the risk of a much larger loss. This is formally described as being risk seeking for gains and risk averse for losses. Third, people are disproportionately concerned about small gains compared to big gains, and about small losses compared to big losses. That is, small changes from the status quo have greater subjective effects than the same increment would have further from the reference point. More formally, the loss function is convex (small losses are more aversive than a linear function of their absolute magnitude) and the gain function is concave (small gains loom larger than a linear function of their material magnitude). Visually, the utility function—the relation between expected value and utility—is a non-linear, somewhat "S" shaped curve.

Applying prospect theory to social relations suggests that dispassionately reasoning people will tend to make choices that undermine social relationships. Being more concerned about losses than gains means that people will be averse to all kinds of reciprocity. This is especially obvious with respect to the in-kind reciprocity and turn-taking of Equality Matching relationships: People more concerned about avoiding losses than they are about acquiring gains will be unwilling to take turns, reluctant to give a present in return for a comparable present or to host a dinner party in the expectation of being invited back, and resistant to doing a favor in return for a comparable favor. In such exchanges what people have to give up looms larger than what they get, even if they get it immediately. If the reciprocity is delayed, hyperbolic discounting makes the problem worse. Loss aversion is also likely to make people resist dividing something equally, contributing equal shares, or doing equal tasks, because what they give up feels greater than what they get, although the objective quantities are equal. Other forms of relationship are also undermined by loss aversion for similar reasons. For example, when Market Pricing requires investment, it will be difficult for people to pay (suffer a loss) in order to gain returns that are objectively larger—quite aside from the discounting of future returns.

These problems are further compounded by the overvaluing of small changes compared to larger increments, described in prospect theory as the convexity of the gain function and the concavity of the loss function. Prospect theory predicts that people will be unwilling to participate in relationships if they have to look beyond small costs or gains to consider the aggregate effects of their actions. Sustaining relationships (the big gain) typically requires a willingness to forgo many small gains. But subjectively, small gains are more than additive compared to large gains: people prefer a series of separate small gains more than a single large gain that equals the sum of the small ones. People are tempted to eat all the cookies in the cookie jar, or spend most of the money in your joint checking account, because each cookie and each purchase looms subjectively large. That is, prospect theory implies that people won't be motivated by the big picture—people will be concerned with the small day to day gains and losses, to the neglect of the big issues that are at stake.

Conversely, people are much more averse to a series of separate small losses than they are to one big loss that equals the sum of the small losses. This means that dispassionately rational people will generally not be willing to incur the small costs of making the small personal sacrifices that sustain relationships because, taken separately one by one, they loom disproportionately large in comparison to the value of the relationships. People will accept the prospect of a big loss if they can avoid many smaller losses that materially add up to the amount of the big loss. If you want to sustain a marriage or the trust of your platoon you must incur many small losses in order to avoid the much bigger ultimate loss of the relationship itself or the cost of a severe sanction such as divorce or loss of the support of your fellow soldiers in the crunch. If you want to sustain any cooperative endeavor, you have to incur a lot of small costs: you have to pitch in when you'd rather goof off, to do a lot of small chores, get out of bed and get to work when you'd rather sleep, pass up all sorts of other opportunities to act selfishly, share resources in small increments, and undergo small privations. Prospect theory predicts that you won't be willing to incur a lot of small costs even if the one big befit of doing so far outweighs the sum of the costs. This does not bode well for social relations.

The over-valuing of small changes from the baseline will make people unwilling to engage in the courtship that is necessary to establish many important social relationships. Courtship requires making many small efforts—paying small costs—in pursuit of the big 'payoff' of the relationship that can ultimately be created. But prospect theory tells us that people will undervalue the great objective expected utility of the relationship and overvalue the small costs of the actions required.

The third thesis of prospect theory is that subjective evaluation of the risk of losses is not symmetrical with evaluation of uncertain gains: people choose risky large gains whose expected value is smaller than a certain gain, but prefer a certain small loss over a large risk whose expected magnitude is smaller.[3] So, for example, many people choose one chance in a million of winning $2,000,000 in preference to a certain $5 (which is why people buy lottery tickets). But most people prefer a certain loss of $5 over one chance in a million of losing $2,000,000 (which is why people buy insurance). This is what is called risk seeking with regard to gains, and risk aversion with regard to losses. Hence a person who could accept the small but sure gains of a subordinate position is likely to take excessive risks in pursuit of the large gain of winning a top position. Similarly, a person who could share a resource with the assurance of getting a modest portion for himself may prefer the high risk entailed in trying to keep the whole resource for himself. Conversely, prospect theory suggests that a person trapped in an exploitive relationship in which the other person cheats or imposes other losses will indefinitely accept these consistent, predictable, small costs, instead of facing the small probability of a severe reprisal for leaving it.

In short, prospect theory's discoveries about human preferences suggest that people will be unable to do what is necessary to sustain meaningful, mutually rewarding, adaptively functional social relationships.

In sum, dispassionate reasoners often are unaware of the social consequences of their actions, do not fully appreciate other's perspectives, fall into the pitfall of reasoning toward their desires, underestimate the risks of appealing and beneficial actions, do not take base rates into account when thinking about their own chances, treat small probabilities as impossibilities, vastly underestimate compound probabilities, over estimate their own control over outcomes, do not appreciate the geometric spread of gossip, hyperbolically discount future sanctions and benefits, overvalue present gains (so they are tempted by immediate desires), overvalue small gains compared to large ones,

---

3.   This discussion simplifies prospect theory, ignoring the interaction between the S-shaped value function and risk seeking or risk aversion. More precisely, people are risk-averse regarding gains involving intermediate probabilities and regarding small probability losses. But people are risk-seeking toward intermediate likelihood of losses and small probability gains. In this respect and others, there is a high probability of large gains from deeper study of the consequences of prospect theory for social relationships.

excessively avoid small losses compared to large ones, take irrational risks in pursuit of gains, and are excessively concerned to avoid risks of large losses.

These limitations of human reasoning and motivation make people prone to give in to temptations to violate important social relationships, and incline people to shirk crucial duties. The result of all of these factors is that neither learning from personal experience nor dispassionate human reasoning can sustain long term social relationships. Learning from available social feedback, utilizing human reasoning processes, and temporally discounted subjective preferences all consistently lead to the choice to defect, cheat, or enjoy immediate gratifications that jeopardize long term social relationships. Dispassionate reasoners will not make the effort to engage in and sustain social relationships. So how do humans achieve the self-control necessary to sustain enduring social relationships that are mutually meaningful, satisfying, and rewarding? Conversely, what do rational FTD patients lack—what is missing, making it so disappointing and unsatisfying to relate to them?

### Social Motives and Moral Emotions are Essential Proxies for the Value of Social Relationships

Even if learning were feasible and people were rational, action depends on having goals for reasoning and rewards that shape learning. Humans, like all organisms, require proximate motivational representations of their adaptive and functional needs. These motives must be given determinate form by cultural transmission, individual experience, and social processes. Humans depend on social relations to live and prosper, so social relationships must be among their fundamental goals and reinforcers. That is what social motives and moral emotions are.

In the dominant theory, people engage in social relationships instrumentally, as rational means to non-social ends. In most versions of this theory, emotions are disruptive forces that interfere with rational pursuit of goals. So the dominant paradigm in the social and behavioral sciences predicts that people should function just fine without emotions. But in fact, people do *not* think about their relationships like economists, behaviorists, direct fitness maximizers, or sociopaths—people feel like lovers, parents, warriors, poets and penitents. The principal forces that direct human social conduct are emotions such as love, affection, loyalty, embarrassment, shame, guilt, jealousy, envy, sorrow, and loneliness. These social emotions are proxies representing the long run benefits of relationships; these emotions provide the moment-to-moment, on-line guidance people need in order to sustain functional relationships. Social emotions are proximate motivational signals of the adaptive, cultural, or personal value of relationships. FTD patients lack these motivational proxies for the long-term value of relationships: they don't experience moral emotions or social needs.

If social emotions are motives that represent the social consequences of present action, then emotions must be proxies for the basic systemic states of relationships. That is, a functional analyses suggests there must be

1. **Appetitive** emotions that motivate people to seek to form relationships. These emotions are signals of the need for relationships. Loneliness is an obvious example.

2. **Consumatory** emotions that are rewards for forming and sustaining relationships. An example is the sense of loving oneness, evidently mediated by oxytocin.

3. **Self-controlling** emotions that motivate the efforts to perform obligations and refrain from satisfying non-social motives that would lead to violations of social relationships. The essence of self-controlling emotions is an aversive reaction at the prospect of violating a relationships, signaling to oneself the dangerous consequences. Embarrassment and shame are examples.

4. **Reparative** emotions that motivate actions to redress one's own violations. For example, guilt, remorse. Self-controlling and reparative emotions are closely linked and may overlap.

5. **Punitive** emotions that motivate punishing others for their transgressions against oneself and against valued others. Vengeful anger is a prototype.

6. **Relinquishment** emotions that motivate withdrawal from deleterious relationships. Hatred is a prototype; consider also some kinds of social disgust.

7. **Loss** emotions that signal to oneself the vulnerability resulting from a partner's departure or death. Mournful sadness is an obvious example.

Functionally, at least some of these seven types of emotions should be specific to each of the four relational models theory (Fiske 1991, 2002). That is, the appetitive need for Communal Sharing should be distinct from the appetitive needs specific to each of the other three fundamental relationships. Likewise, the consumatory emotions of Authority Ranking should be distinct from the rewards specific to the other emotions. Loss emotions may also be specific to the type of relationship. It is not clear whether we should expect distinct self-controlling, reparative, punitive, and relinquishment emotions for each relational model, or whether all that is functionally required is simply that the relevant emotion be oriented to the specific acts and partners. In any case, while based on universal proclivities, human emotions must be tuned to the relationships that are culturally important in the community in which a person grew up. And of course social emotions reflect some of the particulars of each person's relational history and current circumstances.

In all their variants, social motives and moral emotions function as current representations of the future value of social relationships. Thus social motives and moral emotions circumvent reasoning biases and barriers to learning that would otherwise result in maladaptive actions jeopardizing valuable social relationships. The social blindness, heuristics and biases summarized above have little effect on responses to present circumstances; they do not interfere with effective current action to deal with salient, immediately impinging factors in the current situation, including others' directives, requests, and perceptible responses to one's own actions. What the social blindness, biases, and heuristics impede is prudent action to assure the sustainability of social relationships in the long run. To work around these cognitive limitations, people need social motives and moral emotions that are present proxies for future social relational benefits.

Female birds and mammals (and in some species, males and other kin) have evolved "motives" and "emotions" to feed their offspring, defend them, and keep them warm. These motives and emotions are necessary to drive this adaptive behavior, and to counteract basic non-social "emotions" such as hunger, fear, and pain that would otherwise result in the neglect and death of offspring. Adaptive behavior in humans requires analogous emotions and motives, and humans depend on many other social relationships, as well. Humans need motives and emotions to seek, sustain, avoid defecting from, repair, sanction, give up when necessary, and deal with the loss of each of the types of relationships that is important for human survival and reproduction.

Gradually losing social motives and moral emotions, FTD patients no longer make the effort necessary to sustain relationships. They no longer try to control their basic, non-social motives and emotions, and they cease to try to fulfill their social obligations. For quite a while after the onset of FTD, patients continue to be responsive to some immediate social cues, especially directives, and they maintain their memory, knowledge, learning capacities, and reasoning. But FTD begins when social motives and moral emotions fade away and they have only dispassionate rationality to rely on.

FTD is not the only disorder that is characterized by deficient social motives and moral emotions. Others include psychopathy, antisocial personality disorder (PD), schizoid PD, major depression, and forms of schizophrenia. Using behavioral measures as well as parental reports, G.M. Fiske found that young children with autism are less socially motivated than typical children (G.M. Fiske 2008). Conversely, there are disorders in which specific social motives and moral emotions seem to be dysfunctionally intense, including Williams syndrome, paranoid PD, schizotypal PD, borderline PD, histrionic PD, narcissistic PD, and dependent PD. Haslam and colleagues have found that excessive or insufficient dispositions to constitute specific relational models are involved in many of these disorders and predict vulnerability to others (Allen *et al.* 2005; Haslam 2004b; Haslam *et al.* 2002). Measurement of social motives and moral emotions is difficult, however, because people—especially people with some of these disorders—often cannot accurately judge their own sentiments or report them in ways that are interpersonally comparable. Hence to assess social motives and moral emotions in these disorders it will be necessary to use the combination of methods described above. Then we will need to understand what distinguishes these disorders. We need to understand, for example, why FTD patients are generally less manipulative and less violent that psychopaths.

With this framework, we can fruitfully return to the question of why FTD patients lack insight: why do they not realize that they have become amoral and asocial? The simplest theory that accounts for this is that one's own actions and others' reactions are linked to one's representation of the self through social motives and moral emotions. That is, the self is not simply a direct representation of memories of perceptions of social interactions; a crucial facet of what is represented is memory of one's own emotional reactions to those social interactions with respect to one's social motives. Thus the self is an experiential distillate of remembered emotional experiences of social relationships. When a person stops experiencing these emotions and motives, the self fossilizes.

Studying FTD is extraordinarily informative about the self, social and non-social emotions and motives, reasoning and rationality, and social relationships. In particular, FTD patients show us how dispassionate, heuristically rational actors behave. They show us that social motives and moral emotions are necessary to sustain meaningful, trusting, functional social relationships. Human reasoning, with its heuristics, biases, and blind spots, is insufficient: dispassionately rational actors are social failures. Fortunately, most humans are passionate.

## References

Ainslie, G., and N. Haslam.

1992 Hyperbolic discounting. In *Choice over Time,* edited by G. Lowenstein and J. Elster, 57–92. New York: Russell Sage Foundation.

Allen, N.B., A. Semadar and N. Haslam.

2005 Relationship patterns associated with dimensions of vulnerability to psychopathology. *Cognitive Therapy and Research* 29: 737–750. DOI: 10.1007/s10608-005-4607-6

Armor, D.A. and S.E. Taylor.

2002 When predictions fail: The dilemma of unrealistic optimism. In *Heuristics and Biases: The Psychology of Intuitive Judgment,* edited by T. Gilovich, D.W. Griffin, and D. Kahneman, 334–347. New York: Cambridge University Press.

Bar-Hillel, M.

1973 On the subjective probability of compound events. *Organizational Behavior and Human Performance* 9: 396–406.

Beer, J.S., E.A. Heerey, D. Keltner, D. Scabini and R.T. Knight.

2003 The regulatory function of self-conscious emotion: Insights from patients with orbitofrontal damage. *Journal of Personality and Social Psychology* 85: 594–604.

Boone, K.B., B.L. Miller, A. Lee, N. Berman, D. Sherman and D.T. Stuss.

1999 Neuropsychological patterns in right versus left frontotemporal dementia. *Journal of the International Neuropsychological Society* 5: 616–622.

Campbell, D.T. and D.W. Fiske.

1959 Convergent and discriminant validation by the multitrait-multimethod matrix. *Psychological Bulletin* 56: 81–105

Carter, C.S., A.C. DeVries, S.E. Taymans, R.L. Roberts, J.R. Williams and L.L. Getz.

1999 Peptides, steroids, and pair bonding. In *The Integrative Neurobiology of Affiliation,* edited by C.S. Carter, I.I. Lederhendler and B. Kirkpatrick, 169–181. Cambridge, MA: MIT Press.

Clark, A. W., C.L. White, H.J. Manz, I.M. Parhad, B. Curry, P.J. Whitehouse, J. Lehmann, and J.T. Coyle

1986 Primary degenerative dementia without Alzheimer pathology. *Canadian Journal of Neurological Science* 13: 462–470.

Cohen, J. and C.E.M. Hansel.

1958 The nature of decisions in gambling. *Acta Psychologica* 13: 357–370.

Cohen, J., E.I. Chesnick and D. Haran.

1982 Evaluation of compound probabilities in sequential choice. In *Judgment Under Uncertainty: Heuristics and Biases,* edited by D. Kahneman, P. Slovic and A. Tversky, 355–358. Cambridge: Cambridge University Press.

de Bono, M.

2003 Molecular approaches to aggregation behavior and social attachment. *Journal of Neurobiology* 54: 78–92.

Depue, R.A. and J.V. Morrone-Strupinsky.

2005 A neurobehavioral model of affiliative bonding: Implications for conceptualizing a human trait of affiliation. *Behavior and Brain Sciences* 28: 313–349.

Dunning, D., D.W. Griffin, J. Milojkovic. and L. Ross.

1990 The overconfidence effect in social prediction. *Journal of Personality and Social Psychology* 58: 568–581.

Fishoff, B., P. Slovic, S. Lichtenstein, S. Reid and B. Coombs.

1978 How safe is safe enough? A psychometric study of attitudes towards technological risks and benefits. *Policy Sciences* 9: 127–152.

Fiske, A.P.

1991 *Structures of Social Life: The Four Elementary Forms of Human Relations.* New York: Free Press.

2002 Moral emotions provide the self-control needed to sustain social relationships. *Self and Identity* 1: 169–175.

2004 Four modes of constituting relationships: Consubstantial assimilation; space, magnitude, time and force; concrete procedures; abstract symbolism. In *Relational Models Theory: A Contemporary Overview*, edited by N. Haslam, 61–146. Mahwah, NJ: Erlbaum.

Fiske, A.P. and N. Haslam.

2005 The four basic social bonds: Structures for coordinating interaction. In *Interpersonal Cognition*, edited by M. Baldwin, 267–298. New York: Guilford.

Fiske, D.W.

1982 Convergent–discriminant validation in measurements and research strategies. In *Forms of Validity in Research*, edited by D. Brinbirg and L.H. Kidder, 77–92. San Francisco, CA: Jossey-Bass.

Fiske, G.M.

2008 Exploring Motivation for Social Interaction in Children with Autism. Unpublished PhD dissertation, Department of Communication Sciences and Disorders, Northwestern University.

Frank, R.H.

1988 *Passions Within Reason: The Strategic Role of the Emotions.* New York: W.W. Norton.

Gallistel, C.R. and J. Gibbon.

2000 Time, rate, and conditioning. *Psychological Review* 107: 289–344.

Gigerenzer, G. and R. Hertwig.

1999 The 'conjunction fallacy' revisited: How intelligent inferences look like reasoning errors. *Journal of Behavioral Decision Making* 12: 275–305.

Goodwin, C., ed.

2003 *Conversation and Brain Damage.* Oxford: Oxford University Press.

Goodwin, C., M.H. Goodwin and D. Olsher.

2002 Producing sense with nonsense syllables: Turn and sequence in the conversations of a man with severe aphasia. In *The Language of Turn and Sequence,* edited by B. Fox, C. Ford and S. Thompson, 56-80. Oxford: Oxford University Press.

Grewen, K.M., S.S. Girdler, J. Amico and K.C. Light.

2005 Effects of partner support on resting oxytocin, cortisol, norepinephrine, and blood pressure before and after warm partner contact. *Psychosomatic Medicine* 67: 531–538.

Haslam, N., ed.

2004a *Relational Models Theory: A Contemporary Overview.* Mahwah, NJ: Erlbaum.

2004b A relational approach to the personality disorders. In *Relational Models Theory: A Contemporary Overview,* edited by N. Haslam, 335–362. Mahwah, NJ: Erlbaum.

Haslam, N., T. Reichert and A.P. Fiske.

2002 Aberrant social relations in the personality disorders. *Psychology and Psychotherapy: Theory, Research and Practice* 75: 19–31.

Insel, T.R., and L.J. Young.

2001 The neurobiology of attachment. *Nature Reviews Neuroscience* 2: 129–136.

Jagust, W.J., B.R. Reed, J.P. Scab, J.H. Kramer and T.F. Budinger.

1989 Clinical-physiologic correlates of Alzheimer's disease and frontal lobe dementia. *American Journal of Physiologic Imaging* 4: 89–96.

Kahneman, D. and A. Tversky.

1979) Prospect theory: An analysis of decision under risk. *Econometrica* 47: 263–291.

Kendrick, K.M.

2000 Oxytocin, motherhood and bonding. *Experimental Physiology* 85: 111S–124S.

Kunda, Z.

1990 The case for motivated reasoning. *Psychological Bulletin* 108: 480–498.

1999 *Social Cognition: Making Sense of People.* Cambridge, MA: MIT Press.

Langer, E.J.

1975 The illusion of control. *Journal of Personality and Social Psychology* 32: 311–328.

The Lund and Manchester Groups.

1994 Clinical and neuropathological criteria for frontotemporal dementia. *Journal of Neurology, Neurosurgery, and Psychiatry* 57: 416–418.

Matthiesen, A.S., A.B. Ransjo-Arvidson, E. Nissen and K. Uvnäs-Moberg.

2001 Postpartum maternal oxytocin release by newborns: Effects of infant hand massage and sucking. *Birth-Issues in Perinatal Care* 28: 13–19.

McKhann, G.M., M.S. Albert, M. Grossman, B. Miller, D. Dickson and J.Q. Trojanowski.

2001 Clinical and pathological diagnosis of frontotemporal dementia: Report of the work group on frontotemporal dementia and pick's disease. *Archives of Neurology* 58: 1803–1809.

Mendez, M.

2006 What frontotemporal dementia reveals about the neurobiological basis of morality. *Medical Hypotheses* 67: 411–418.

Mendez, M., E. Anderson and J.S. Shapira.

2005 An investigation of moral judgment in frontotemporal dementia. *Cognitive and Behavioral Neurology* 18: 193–197.

Mendez, M.F., A.K. Chen, J.S. Shapira and B.L. Miller.

2005 Acquired sociopathy and frontotemporal dementia. *Dementia and Geriatric Cognitive Disorders* 20: 99–104.

Mendez, M.F., M. Cherrier, K.M. Perryman, N. Pachana, B.L. Miller and J.L. Cummings.

1996 Frontotemporal dementia vs. Alzheimer's disease: Differential cognitive features. *Neurology* 47: 1189–1194.

Mendez, M. F., and J. L. Cummings

2003 *Dementia: A Clinical Approach,* 3rd edition. Philadelphia: Butterworth-Heienmann.

Mikesell, L.

2009a Exploring the Language and Social Behavior of Frontotemporal Dementia: How Patients and Caregivers Manage Interaction. Unpublished Ph.D. Dissertation, Department of Applied Linguistics and TESL, UCLA.

2009b Conversational practices of a frontotemporal dementia patient and his interlocutors. *Research on Language and Social Interaction* 42(2): 135–162.

Miller, B.L., W.W. Seeley, P. Mychack, H.J. Rosen, I. Mena and K. Boone.

2001 Neuroanatomy of the self: Evidence from patients with frontotemporal dementia. *Neurology* 57: 817–821.

Mychack, P., J.H. Kramer, K.B. Boone and B.L. Miller.

2001 The influence of right frontotemporal dysfunction on social behavior in frontotemporal dementia. *Neurology* 56 (11 Supplement 4): S11–5

Neary, D., J.S. Snowden, L. Gustafson, U. Passant, D. Stuss, S. Black, M. Freedman, A. Kertesz, P.H. Robert, M. Albert, K. Boone, B.L. Miller, J. Cummings, and D.F. Benson.

1998 Frontotemporal lobar degeneration: A consensus on clinical diagnostic criteria. *Neurology* 51(6): 1546–1554.

Panksepp, J.

1998 *Affective Neuroscience: The Foundations of Human and Animal Emotions.* New York: Oxford University Press.

Passant, U., C. Elfgren, E. Englund, and L. Gustafson.

2005 Psychiatric symptoms and their psychosocial consequences in frontotemporal dementia. *Alzheimer Disease and Associated Disorders* 19: 15–18 (supplement 1).

Rule, R.R., A.P. Simamura and R.T. Knight.

2002 Orbitofrontal cortex and dynamic filtering of emotional stimuli. *Cognitive, Affective, and Behavioral Neuroscience* 2: 264–270.

Slovic, P., B. Fischoff and S. Lichtenstein.

1982 Facts versus fears: Understanding perceived risk. In *Judgment Under Uncertainty: Heuristics and Biases,* edited by D. Kahneman, P. Slovic and A. Tversky, 463–489. Cambridge: Cambridge University Press.

Slovic, P., D.G. MacGregor, T. Malmfors and I.F.H. Purchase.

1999 *Influence of Affective Processes on Toxicologists' Judgments of Risk* (Report No. 99–2) Eugene, OR: Decision Research.

Snowden, J.S., D. Bathgate, A. Varma, A. Blackshaw, Z. C. Gibbons, and D. Neary.

2001 Distinct behavioural profiles in frontotemporal dementia and semantic dementia. *Journal of Neurology, Neurosurgery and Psychiatry* 70(3): 323-332.

Stivers, T.

2005 Modified repeats: One method for asserting primary rights from second position. *Research on Language and Social Interaction* 38: 131–158.

Tversky, A. and D. Kahneman.

1982 Evidential impact of base rates. In *Judgment Under Uncertainty: Heuristics and Biases,* edited by D. Kahneman, P. Slovic and A. Tversky, 153–160. Cambridge: Cambridge University Press.

1983 Extensional versus intuitive reasoning: The conjunction fallacy in probability judgment. *Psychological Review* 90: 293–315.

1991 Loss aversion in riskless choice: a reference-dependent model. *The Quarterly Journal of Economics* 106: 1039–1061.

UCSF documentary cited in Mikesell 2009a. Formerly at http://www.memory.ucsf.edu/Documentary_Site/film.html, but this link was later broken.

Uvnäs-Moberg, K.

1998 Oxytocin may mediate the benefits of positive social interaction and emotions. *Psychoneuroendocrinology* 23: 819–835.

Weinstein, N.

1989 Perceptions of personal susceptibility to harm. In *Psychological Approaches to the Primary Prevention of Acquired Immune Deficiency Syndrome,* edited by V. Mays, G. Albee and F. Schneider, 142–167. Newbury Park, CA: Sage.

Young, L.J., M.M. Lim, B. Gingrich and T.R. Insel.

2001 Cellular mechanisms of social attachment. *Hormones and Behavior* 40: 133–138.

Zald, D.H. and S.W. Kim.

2001 The orbitofrontal cortex. In *The Frontal Lobes and Neuropsychiatric Illness,* edited by S.P. Salloway, P.F. Malloy and J.D. Duffy, 33–70. Washington, DC: American Psychiatric Press.

**9**

# Brain, Language, Society: Where FTD Has Led Us

John H. Schumann

Since 1987, the Applied Linguistics program at UCLA has been training students in neurobiology in order to understand how the brain operates in language acquisition and use. The students' linguistic focus centers on conversation analysis and discourse analysis because we believe that it is important to understand the dyadic brain. Psychology and neuroscience generally have examined the isolated brain in clinical and laboratory settings. But it is reasonable to assume that the brain evolved to interact with other brains and the interactional orientation of conversational analysis and discourse analysis thus provides a behavioral window on brain–brain interaction. Currently we have a group of students who are examining the conversational interaction of patients with frontotemporal dementia (FTD). FTD is a progressive degeneration of the frontal lobes and also sometimes of the anterior temporal lobes. The frontal lobes are the most rostral part of the brain and seem to subserve social knowledge and skill, as well as reasoning about social and personal issues (Damasio 1994).

Research by Damasio (1994) indicates that patients with damage to the ventromedial part of the pre-frontal cortex have difficulty maintaining socially appropriate behavior and also have difficulty generating decisions that are in their best interest. He argues that prefrontal damage severs the connection between the brain and the body proper. Normal individuals confronting a stimulus situation get feedback from their autonomic nervous systems, endocrine systems, and musculoskeletal systems. This feedback from the body constitutes an emotion that is perceived by the brain as a feeling. The feeling (positive or negative) helps an individual choose among possible courses of action. The research on prefrontal damage has generally reported that FTD patients have normal language. However those of us who were working on the social aspects of language felt that the difficulties prefrontal patients had with socially appropriate behavior were bound to be reflected in their speech. In normal conversational interactions one has to make personal and social decisions concerning appropriateness on a moment to moment, word by word, pause by pause basis. Therefore, we hypothesized that people with prefrontal damage particularly in the ventromedial and orbitofrontal areas would have deficits in language pragmatics (Schumann 1999). One way to explore this hypothesis would be to conduct conversation analyses ordinary, outside-of-the-clinic of normal interaction between FTD patients and members of their family.

The decision-making that is carried out via the PFC seems to be the outcome of stimulus appraisal. Following on the work of Scherer (1984), Schumann (1997, 1999) and others, we have argued that the bodily state would be the result of evaluations of stimulus situations made along several parameters: novelty, pleasantness, goal or need significance, coping potential, and self and social image. A novelty appraisal determines whether the stimulus is new or whether it has been experienced previously. Novelty can be appraised positively or negatively. A stimulus might be seen as novel and therefore interesting or as so unusual that it is threatening. An evaluation along the goal/need dimension determines whether the stimulus situation is conducive to achieving one's goal or satisfying one's needs. Coping potential refers to the individual's determination of whether or not he/she is capable of dealing with the physical or psychological consequences of the situation. Appraisals on the self and social image dimension determine how engaging in the stimulus situation would affect the individual's notion of his or her ideal self or how it would affect the evaluation of the individual by significant others. These five dimensions of stimulus appraisal contribute to the decision making carried out via the prefrontal cortex.

Stimulus appraisal is embedded in more general processes of social cognition and theory of mind. In order to produce pragmatically appropriate speech, interlocutors have to engage their stimulus appraisal mechanisms to make hypotheses about each other's intentionality. That is, the interlocutors must be able to assess each other's needs, desires, emotions, feelings, and cognitions and to appraise their emotional and motivational relevance. Thus,

> in normal social interaction we make judgments about our interlocutors' intentions, emotions, beliefs, and behaviors. We appraise these judgments according to their novelty (i.e., conformity or discrepancy with what is expected), pleasantness, and how they might challenge our ability to cope with this situation. In addition, we assess judgments about our interlocutor's

state of mind and behavior according to whether they foster our goals and according to whether they are enhancing of our self and social image. On the basis of these appraisals, we decide (consciously or unconsciously) to be polite or rude, aggressive or calm, direct or indirect, loud or quiet, clear or vague, truthful or untruthful, dominant or submissive, and we choose our phonology, prosody, grammar and lexicon accordingly.

(Schumann 1999, 294).

This decision-making process, we assumed, would be compromised in FTD patients and as a result, their conversational interactions would reflect that deficit.

We know that the pre-frontal cortex matures slowly and does not complete its development until late in the second decade of life (Sowell, Thompson, Holmes, Batth, Jernigan and Toga 1999; Casey *et al.* 2005). The work on FTD illustrates that this part of the brain is also vulnerable to degeneration. Damasio (1994) has demonstrated that people with injuries to the ventromedial prefrontal cortex retain their knowledge of the rules for appropriate social behavior, but they are unable to implement them. He suggests that the ventromedial prefrontal cortex is part of a neural system that mediates socialization, enculturation, and education. Based on the FTD research, we might include the temporal poles in this system. As we have seen, the discourse of FTD patients is frequently characterized by perseverative speech where the patient repeats himself or by substantially depressed verbal output in which the patient simply does not respond. Recent research on the most anterior part of the prefrontal cortex, the frontal pole, offers an explanation for these behaviors. The frontal polar cortex maintains representations of behaviors, tasks, and responses that have to be postponed while another task is being carried out. It then allows the selection of a pending task when the previous one has been completed. It can do this without external cues. There may be several pending tasks, behaviors, or responses that have to be held in memory and the choice which to engage in is not necessarily fixed. The selection of the appropriate response or behavior may be known only milliseconds before it must be generated, and then within another few milliseconds, the response chosen may require that a decision be made about the choice of a subsequent response (Koechlin and Hyafil 2007).

Merlin Donald has characterized these mental operations in similar ways.

In order to follow [a] conversation, we must keep the ideas of the various participants in separate areas of memory, properly labeled and updated. The conversation is loaded with information, feeling tones, and clashes. Even the humor and the personality conflicts must be noted and remembered. We place a huge load on conscious capacity when we are faced with such a challenge, especially such an unpredictable one. In technical terms, we draw on our finite conscious capacity. A complex conversation can push that capacity to its limits because it generates novel, rich, and meaningful memory material, highly changeable from moment to moment, as the conversation shifts from topic to topic,…and speaker to speaker. It is an incredible achievement that despite this complexity, a conversation usually coheres in memory as a single unified episode. (2001, 49)

In addition to the prefrontal cortex, the neural system extends to the amygdala (Schumann 1997; Schumann *et al.* 2004), the insula (Craig 2002), the retrosplenial area (Ullsperger 2008) and the body proper (Damasio 1994). Damasio (1994) has shown that the last component includes the autonomic nervous system, the endocrine system, and the musculoskeletal system. In fact, he argues that the emotions are generated in these parts of the body and are then communicated to the brain as feelings that help guide social decision-making and behavior. We might also include in the system Porges' (2003) notion of the polyvagal circuit, most especially the segment which modulates social engagement (special visceral efferent pathways which control head and face muscles and a visceromotor component which regulates the heart and lungs). It would appear that people with prefrontal damage have a disruption in information flow between the brain and the body (the peripheral nervous system). Therefore, this malady illustrates the advisability of thinking in terms of the nervous system, not just in terms of the brain.

The research on the prefrontal cortex illustrates the exquisite coordination between society and biology. The prefrontal cortex is actually molded by social interaction (Schore 1994); it evolved to subserve social experiences first by being shaped by experience, incorporating it as knowledge, and then by governing an individual's social behavior via that knowledge. Society builds each person's prefrontal cortex, and then the prefrontal cortex guides the persons' social interactions. Because the prefrontal cortex is built by experience in the world, and because people's early experience varies from excellent, to adequate, to toxic, society has had to evolve practices and institutions to construct the system, to support it when it is challenged, and to remediate it when it is damaged. Let's examine some of the manifestation of these "external prefrontal cortices."

I had a relative who was doing very poorly in high school and was frequently getting into trouble with school authorities and even the police. When he was a senior, he took a set of aptitude tests for the Navy. He scored very high and the recruiting office made extraordinary efforts to get him to enlist—even to the extent that they showed up at his home on the day of his math final and drove him to school. He ultimately joined and remained for four years. The intense discipline and training he received during this time, I would suggest, may have developed his prefrontal cortex, providing him with the ability to self regulate, to focus, to think ahead, to respect authority, and to interact in socially appropriate ways. When he left the Navy, he attended a prestigious engineering college and now runs his own company. I would suggest that for much of the four years of his service, the military acted as an external prefrontal cortex providing, through external regulation, the training and experience necessary for the prefrontal cortex to develop circuits required for personal descending control. The idea that military training and experience can produce mature young men and women has been around for a long time. Here I am just pointing out what may be the biological response to that training.

Several of the articles in this volume illustrate the FTD patients' need for external regulation to negotiate their everyday lives. It is as though their caregivers are acting as auxiliary prefrontal cortices to guide them in correct social behavior. This is manifest in caregivers' modulation of patients' inappropriate behavior and their attempts to socially engage the patients with apathetic variant of FTD (see for example Mikesell 2009).

Mikesell (this volume) examined how caregivers try to manage an FTD patient's perseverative behavior. She noted that they employ three strategies: reasoning, distracting, and physically directing. Avineri (this volume) studied an FTD patient's difficulties with "insight" about her problems. Her analysis indicates that this patient is unaware of her difficulties, but she is aware that her caregivers believe she has problems. Therefore, when asked by a doctor, for example, whether she has any difficulties, she suggests that he ask the caregiver. So although she is unaware of her own internal state, she can call on another person to fill in the gap. Smith (this volume) demonstrated that FTD patients perform better in conversation if the discourse is about them. This self-bias skews normal conversational interaction and requires an external regulation to ameliorate it. The only way to adequately discover and display the patients' discoursal deficits and their caregivers attempts to ameliorate them is through a microanalysis of natural interaction provided by conversational analysis. Both casual observation and psycholinguistic testing that is typical of clinical assessment would miss the subtlety and pervasiveness of the interactional deficits.

Joaquin (this volume) demonstrated the efforts parents and caregivers make to socialize children to the standards of behavior expected by society. In her chapter, we saw socialization taking place in the home and in preschools in several cultures. Here we see parents and caregivers acting as external prefrontal cortices, but we might also hypothesize that such external control and guidance is provided by societal institutions such as scouts, sports teams, musical training, religious education and the discipline imposed by school requirements and routines.

As we pointed out, the prefrontal cortex and its associated regions respond to the environment, and environments vary. Therefore, where adequate socialization has not been provided or where it has not been successful, there are other institutions that intervene—legal systems such as the police, probation programs, and prisons. The medical profession via mental-health programs also exists as a societal institution that intervenes to ameliorate misfires in socialization. Therapies and pharmacological interventions are available, in part, to remediate problems in self-regulation and social interaction. What this demonstrates is that normal individuals may, at times, require external prefrontal support. In such cases, the problems usually involve difficulties in modulating aspects of descending control and self-regulation. Normal individuals with intact prefrontal cortices can, with therapy, can acquire new neural circuits that override those that are functioning below par. With FTD patients, the circuits have degenerated and new ones cannot be formed. Therefore, modulation of the patients' descending control and self regulation fall on the caregivers.

As stated earlier, socialization practices, in effect, target the prefrontal cortex by directing or modulating decision making processes and the functions associated with it. They build neural circuits in that area, and during the building process, the socialization practices are serving as external prefrontal cortices. Joaquin's chapter illustrates socialization practices in several societies: American, British, Taiwanese, and Japanese. Anthropologists have pointed out that these practices vary across cultures, and the intense overt caregiver-child interaction manifest in industrialized societies does not seem to characterize child rearing in more traditional cultures. In such cultures, young children are often not addressed directly; they are expected to attend to adult interaction and to learn as watchers and listeners, observing and overhearing what the adults want them to learn and know. Of course, this may mean that these children have greater access to adult society than in industrialized cultures. Socialization by observation, imitation, and participation (but with less verbal interaction) implies a strong belief in implicit learning. Joaquin, in Lee *et al.* (2009), shows that children in industrialized societies are active initiators of social interaction. They seek out that interaction, and their motive is to become like their conspecifics. The adults meet them more than halfway in responding to and generating interaction. In traditional societies, it would appear that the adults, by withholding overt guidance and instruction, rely more heavily on the children's "culture-seeking" proclivities (Tizard and Hughes 1998, 14). What this cultural variation demonstrates is that regardless of the manner in which children are socialized, they are still socialized, that the prefrontal cortices can be targeted by a range of socialization practices, and that external prefrontal cortices can take on many forms.

If we conjecture that the child-rearing practices in industrialized societies represent a change or cultural evolution from traditional behavior, we can ask what made the change come about? One possibility is that it resulted from additional leisure time that could be devoted to children. Another possibility is that the change was the product of widespread schooling. School instruction is typically overt, and there is, of course, substantial emphasis on developing verbal acuity and literacy skills. It may be that schooled adults adapted some educational interaction and instructional practices to child-rearing— seeing children as capable of responding to conversational interaction and profiting from it. Additionally, there may have been implicit recognition that children raised in this way did better in school. An education—child rearing feedback loop may have evolved, generating continuity between home and school. Another possibility is that in the move from the extended family to the nuclear family, mothers may have had no other adults to interact with. Therefore, their children could not learn by observing adult interaction. In this situation, mothers may have been forced to interact directly with their children in order for language acquisition and socialization to be successful (Lofstedt, personal communication, Nov. 2008). Once again, these speculations are consonant with the notion that prefrontal cortex development is dependent on socialization, and societies will struggle to find socialization practices that will accomplish this task.

We might also speculate that different socialization practices exist to produce different kinds of people. The extensive and long-term plasticity of the prefrontal cortex and its influence on related areas may have evolved to produce just such variation. In addition, the two-to-three decade openness of the PFC, allows socialization to various kinds of professional training later in life. Different behaviors and styles of language are required in different professional domains (e.g. engineering, law, medicine, academics, business etc.) and the brain must remain responsive to such training which in contemporary society can extend into one's 20s and 30s.

We might refer to the research in this volume as neuroethnography (Numa Markee, personal communication, Mar. 30, 2008). As such it provides two perspectives, that of a patient and that of his or her interlocutor. This interactant-focus reveals what normal people do in conversation when confronting persons whose interactional capacities are deficient. The authors consider the dyad to be the organism that is studied in conversation. In other words, typical clinical focus on the patient alone is only partially revealing. In neuroethnography, the speaker and interlocutor form a single unit. This focus we believe is important for understanding the brain in interaction with other brains.

## References


Casey, B.J., N. Tottenham, C. Liston and S. Durston.

2005 Imaging the developing brain: What have we learned about cognitive development? *Trends in Cognitive Sciences* 9: 104–110.

Craig, A.D.

2002 How do you feel? Interoception: The sense of the physical condition of the body. *Nature Reviews Neuroscience* 3: 655–666.

Damasio, A.R.

1994 *Decartes's Error: Emotion, reason, and the human brain*. New York: G.P. Putnam's Sons.

Donald, M.

2001 *A mind so rare: The evolution of human consciousness*. New York: W.W. Norton.

Koechlin E. and A. Hyafil.

2007 Anterior prefrontal function and the limits of human-decision–making. *Science* 318: 594–597

Lee, N., L. Mikesell, A.D.L. Joaquin, A.W. Mates and J.H. Schumann.

2009 *The interactional instinct: Language evolution and acquisition*. Oxford: Oxford University Press.

Mikesell, L.

2009 Conversational practices of a frontotemporal dementia patient and his interlocutors. *Research on Language and Social Interaction* 42(2): 135–162.

Porges, S.W.

2003 Social Engagement and attachment: A phylogenetic perspective. *Annals of the New York Academy of Sciences* 1008: 31–47.

Scherer, K. R.

1984 Emotion as a multicomponent process: A model and some cross-cultural data. In *Review of personality and social psychology, 5: Emotions, relationships, and health*, edited by P. Shaver, 37–63. Beverly Hills, CA: Sage.

Schore, A.N.

1994 *Affect regulation and the origin of the self: the neurobiology of emotional development*. Hillsdale, NJ: Lawrence Erlbaum Associates.

Schumann, J.H.

1997 *The neurobiology of affect in language*. Boston: Blackwell. (Also published by the journal, *Language Learning*, as a supplement to volume 48, 1997).

1999 A neurobiological basis for decision making in language pragmatics. *Pragmatics & Cognition* 7: 283–311.

Schumann, J.H., S.E. Crowell, N.E. Jones, N. Lee, S.A. Schuchert and L.A. Wood, eds.

2004 *The Neurobiology of Learning: Perspectives from Second Language Acquisition.* Mahwah, NJ: Lawrence Erlbaum Associates.

Sowell, E.R., P.M. Thompson, C.J. Holmes, R. Batth, T.L. Jernigan and A.W. Toga.

1999 Localizing age-related changes in brain structure between childhood and adolescence using statistical parametric mapping. *NeuroImage* 6: 587–597.

Tizard, B. and M.Hughes.

1984 *Young children learning*. Cambridge, MA: Harvard University Press.

Ullsperger, M.

2008 Minding mistakes. *Scientific American Mind* 19: 52–59.

# Appendix A

Consensus guidelines for the clinical diagnosis of frontotemporal dementia (from Neary *et al.* 1998).

Clinical profile: character change and disordered social conduct are the dominant features initially and throughout the disease course.

Core diagnostic features
> Insidious onset and gradual progression
> Early decline in social interpersonal conduct
> Early impairment in regulation of personal conduct
> Early emotional blunting
> Early loss of insight

Supportive diagnostic features
> *Behavioural disorder*
>> Decline in personal hygiene and grooming
>> Mental rigidity and inflexibility
>> Distractibility and impersistence
>> Hyperorality and dietary changes
>> Perseverative and stereotyped behaviour
>> Utilisation behaviour
>
> *Speech and language*
>> Altered speech output: aspontaneity and economy of speech; press of speech
>> Stereotypy of speech
>> Echolalia
>> Perseveration
>> Mutism
>
> *Physical signs*
>> Primitive reflexes
>> Incontinence
>> Akinesia, rigidity and tremor
>> Low and labile blood pressure

*Investigations*

Neuropsychology: significant impairment on frontal lobe tests in the absence of severe amnesia, aphasia, or perceptuospatial disorder

Electroencephalography: normal on conventional electroencephalogram despite clinically evident dementia

Brain imaging (structural or functional): predominant frontal or anterior temporal abnormality

# Appendix B

## Transcription Conventions

Transcription symbols[1]:

| | |
|---|---|
| ? | Rising inonation |
| . | Falling intonation |
| , | Continuing intonation |
| [ | Overlap |
| : | Vowel lengthening, and stretching of sound |
| <u>wo</u>rd | Underlining is used to indicate stress |
| <u>WO</u>rd | Upper case indicates especially loud talk |
| ^ | Rise in pitch |
| ↑ | Rise in pitch |
| ↓ | Fall in pitch |
| hh | Outbreath |
| .hh | Inbreath |
| (.) | Micro pause |
| (0.1) | Silence in tenths of a second |
| (P) | Silence – no measurement |
| ° | Whisper/breathy speech |
| = | Attaches continuous speech |
| - | Speech cut off |
| >> | Speech rushed |
| > < | Faster rate of speech |
| < > | Slower rate of speech |
| ( ) | Uncertain transcription |
| (( )) | Analyst's comment |

---

1. Adapted from Sacks, H., Schegloff, E.A. & Jefferson, G. (1974). A simplest systematics for the organization of turn-taking for conversation. *Language* 50(4): 696–735.

CPSIA information can be obtained at www.ICGtesting.com
Printed in the USA
BVOW08s0938280515

401964BV00003B/14/P